CHOROIDAL AND CILIARY BODY MALIGNANT MELANOMA

Diagnosis and Management

CHOROIDAL AND CILIARY BODY MALIGNANT MELANOMA

Diagnosis and Management

ROBERT N. JOHNSON, M.D.

Retina Research Fund
San Francisco, California

To Jeannie,
Ryan, and Eric

CONTENTS

CHAPTER 3

DIFFERENTIAL DIAGNOSIS   33

CHAPTER 4

HISTOPATHOLOGY   61

CHAPTER 5

NATURAL HISTORY   69

CHAPTER 6

METASTATIC EVALUATION   73

CHAPTER 7

MANAGEMENT: GENERAL CONSIDERATIONS AND THE ROLE OF OBSERVATION   77

CHAPTER 8

ENUCLEATION   83

CHAPTER 9

RADIATION THERAPY   93

CHAPTER 10

ALTERNATIVE TREATMENT MODALITIES   111

A FINAL PERSPECTIVE   119

INDEX   121

The large literature concerning uveal melanoma during the past two decades reflects the rapidly changing concepts concerning its natural course, relationship to melanocytic nevi, diagnosis, and treatment. Prior to the 1960's, the guiding principle regarding diagnosis and treatment of a suspected uveal melanoma was, "when in doubt, take the eye out." Many factors are responsible for the revolutionary changes that have occurred in regard to management of patients with lesions suspected as uveal melanomas.

Three important events that occurred almost simultaneously during the 1960's was the upsurge in interest in ophthalmic pathology by ophthalmology residents, the development of new techniques of binocular indirect ophthalmoscopy and biomicroscopy, and the emergence of techniques of stereo fundus photography and fluorescein angiography. Thanks to the teaching, writing and inspiration provided by Lorenz E. Zimmerman, Michael J. Hogan, and A. Edward Maumenee, and others, as well as the establishment of grant-supported fellowships in ophthalmic pathology, there appeared a new generation of ophthalmologists skilled in microscopic examination of surgical specimens as well as stereoscopic, ophthalmoscopic, and biomicroscopic examination of the ocular fundus. The availability of stereo fundus photographs and fluorescein angiography permitted documentation of not only anatomic but also physiologic changes associated with intraocular tumors. The ability to detect and record precisely serial changes in intraocular tumors, and to make comparisons of the changes with the histopathology of those tumors that were enucleated, soon led to challenges to long held dogma concerning the clinical features, natural course, and cytologic classification of uveal melanoma and nevi, as well as the dictum that prompt enucleation of all suspected melanomas was essential to prevent metastasis. Observation of patients with melanocytic tumors of uncertain growth potential as well as melanomas in patients refusing enucleation demonstrated that many such tumors fail to grow and presumably are nevi or other benign lesions; others grow and do so at a variable, yet generally constant rate; and observation for evidence of growth appears not to influence the rate of metastases. These observations, together with the as yet unsubstantiated theory of Zimmerman

that enucleation may increase rather than decrease the likelihood of metastases, resulted in renewed effort to find new ways short of enucleation to treat patients with uveal melanomas. These include new techniques of using external charged particle radiation, a variety of isotopes for episcleral implants, photocoagulation, local excision, hyperthermia, and photoradiation.

The new methods of clinical examinations and photographic follow-up of tumors coupled with the greater awareness of clinical and histopathologic features of lesions simulating melanoma are major factors that led to marked reduction in the number of eyes enucleated with an incorrect diagnosis of melanoma. Of the recently developed ancillary studies, ultrasonography has been the most helpful in regard to differential diagnosis of uveal melanoma. Other tests such as radiophosphorus ^{32}P uptake, computerized tomography, and magnetic resonance imaging have proved less valuable.

Although we have made significant advances in our ability to accurately diagnose uveal melanoma clinically and to preserve visual function, we are still left with many important, unresolved issues. Does our management of patients with these tumors play a significant role in the mortality caused by the tumors? How safe is it to observe patients for months or years for evidence of growth before giving treatment? Is prompt removal of the eye containing a melanoma the safest form of therapy? What are the relative risks regarding morbidity and metastases associated with the more conservative forms of therapy. The Collaborative Ocular Melanoma Study should provide us with some of these answers.

Dr. Johnson is to be commended for this valuable, comprehensive review and synthesis of the sometimes conflicting opinions regarding findings, diagnostic procedures, and therapeutic recommendations found in the recent literature concerning uveal melanomas. This book will be a valuable resource for medical students, resident physicians, and the practicing ophthalmologist, as well as ocular oncologists.

J. Donald Gass, M.D.

Ophthalmologists, to some extent, have been spoiled by their experience with radiocurable and chemo-curable diseases such as retinoblastoma, rhabdomysarcoma, and the lymphomas. They then are astonished and dismayed to encounter a tumor like malignant melanoma, which does not respond well to any current chemotherapeutic approach. It is important that we learn more about the natural history of pigmented cells in general and specifically, the similarity and differences between skin melanomas and those involving the uvea.

Dr. Johnson has brilliantly outlined the current knowledge of ocular malignant melanoma in this very well-referenced work and has indicated areas of basic knowledge that might be explored to develop new therapeutic approaches.

Cytogenetic studies in melanoma have, to date, not been as revealing as those in some other ocular tumors, and I suspect that malignant melanoma will be reclassified at a molecular level, perhaps with the help of immunology and ultrasound.

There are few individuals that are well-versed in all of the many aspects of melanoma, and the compilation of this body of knowledge puts Dr. Johnson in a very enviable position to make the intellectual connection that can lead to a new attack on this difficult tumor. Dr. Johnson exemplifies the character of a true physician, and I trust that he will be among the leaders of ophthalmology who are confronting this problem.

Robert M. Ellsworth, M.D.

PREFACE

The scientific literature concerning choroidal and ciliary body malignant melanoma is voluminous even if one considers only the past three decades. Several authors have published well-written ocular oncology texts that have included the subject of malignant choroidal melanoma. These texts provide authoritative information but tend to emphasize the authors' experiences and views. Other expert opinions may not be included. The significance of this is particularly relevant for choroidal and ciliary body melanomas on which widely divergent opinions prevail.

This text reviews and consolidates the many varied opinions, observations and research findings of authorities in this field in order to clarify what is known and accepted as fact; to provide insight into clinical research endeavors that may someday provide more answers, diagnostic tests, or treatment options; and to present aspects of the controversies that exist in the field today. This book focuses on the last three decades because of the number of new developments in the field. Unless indicated specifically, choroidal and ciliary body malignant melanoma are referred to as malignant melanoma.

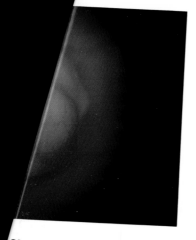
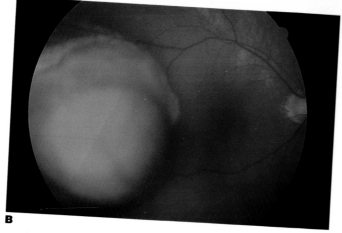

B

Choroidal Malignant Melanoma

blurring of his vision in his right eye for the past year. The visual acuity was 20/32. Note the amelanotic shape. Standardized echography measured the maximal thickness as 7.1 mm.

Although certain features are classic for malignant melanoma, these varied pat- benign and other malignant disorders. e Armed Forces Institute of Pathology ut 20% of eyes enucleated because of a melanoma were misdiagnosed.[36,80] Cur-curacy is better such that a misdiagnosis han 3% of eyes.[2,21,31,76] Several factors have oved accuracy in diagnosis, including more direct ophthalmoscopy, enhanced awareness fused lesions that are sometimes called pseu-**able 1.1**), development of ultrasonography and ography, judicious observation of suspicious d most recently, the application of fine needle sy.[9,10,21,24,28,30,47] These diagnostic modalities do not definitive diagnoses, and exceptions to character-of malignant melanoma ascribed to each of these Nevertheless, reliance on a combination of diagnos-d an understanding of their limitations, can achieve accuracy of about 99%.[19,21,26,57,72,77] diagnosis of malignant melanoma is established, the vantages and disadvantages of several potential treat-ions must be considered. Adding further to the com-f this subject are widely divergent opinions and con-es regarding diagnosis and treatment.[19,21,42,48,62,74,76]

Table 1.1
Pseudomelanomas

Choroidal Nevus	Combined Retinal-RPE[†]
Macular Disciform Scar	Hamartoma
Eccentric Disciform Scar	Luxated Lens
CHRPE[*]	Cavernous Hemangioma of the
Choroidal Hemangioma	Retina
Reactive RPE[†] Hyperplasia	Central Retinal Vein
Melanocytoma	Obstruction
Choroidal Detachment	Reticulum Cell Sarcoma
Hemorrhagic RPE[†] or Retinal	Toxoplasmosis
Detachment	Macular Pucker
Vitreous Hemorrhage	Subretinal Granuloma
Rhegmatogenous Retinal	Histoplasmosis
Detachment	RPE[†] or Ciliary Epithelial
Posterior Scleritis	Adenoma
Metastatic Carcinoma	Myopic Chorioretinal
Retinoschisis	Degeneration
Uveal Effusion Syndrome	Retinitis, Viral
Choroidal Osteoma	

[*] CHRPE—Congenital Hypertrophy of Retinal Pigment Epithelium
[†] RPE—Retinal Pigment Epithelial
(Adapted from Shields, JA, Augsburger, JJ, Brown, GC, Stephens, RF: The differential diagnosis of posterior uveal melanoma. Ophthalmology 87:518-522, 1980.)

ACKNOWLEDGMENTS

In reflecting over the time this book has been underway, many people have affected this project directly or indirectly and have provided invaluable assistance for which I am extremely grateful.

First of all, I wish to thank my associates, Drs. Howard Schatz and H. Richard McDonald. Their encouragement, support, and extensive knowledge and expertise make our relationship and association beyond compare. I am very grateful for this unique association, which allows me to share both work and friendship with such compassionate and gifted physicians.

I am indebted to Dr. J. Donald M. Gass, whose tremendous insight and gift for observation and understanding made my fellowship with him an exceptional experience. I am deeply appreciative of Drs. Robert Ellsworth and David Abramson, who shared freely with me their extensive experience, insight and knowledge of ocular oncology during my fellowship with them. I am thankful for Drs. George Blankenship, John Clarkson, Harry Flynn, Don Nicholson, and Karl Olsen, who patiently taught me my skills as a vitreoretinal surgeon. John Hungerford allowed me a rewarding opportunity to share in the considerable ocular oncology experience of St. Bartholomew's and Moorfields hospital. May Dr. Alex Irvine never lose the energy, patience and dedication to resident teaching that provided me a unique experience as a resident at the University of California, San Francisco. Dr. Jerry Shields shared his patients and knowledge with me. Dr. Devron Char first stimulated my interest in tumors.

A special thank you to all of the members of and contributors to the Northern California Section of the Collaborative Ocular Melanoma Study. The commitment, time, energy and contributions of these individuals have made ours a busy oncology center. To: Robert T. Wendel, Robert S. Fantl, Edwin E. Boldrey, Donald E. Roy, Stanley Galas, Michael W. Gaynon, W. James Gealy, John H. Drouilhet, Conor C. O'Malley, Roger D. Griffith, Sterling J. Haidt, Steven C. Johnson, Neil E. Kelly, Thomas C. Salzano, James W. Wells, Arthur W. Allen, Jr., Peter F. Petersen, Otto G. Klein, Arnold J. Smoller, Glynne Couvillion, Stephen D. Miller, Michael P. Teske, Gregory S. Brinton, Roy A. Goodart, Everett Ai, Eric J. Del Piero, Geoffrey V. Cecchi, F. Temple Riekhof, Gregory C. Tesluk, Patrick Coonan, Peter R. Egbert, and Greer Geiger.

Karen Laughlin and Anne Miller, the administrators and coordinators of our oncology center, have given so much of themselves to our patients by providing compassionate support, understanding, and a willing ear; their dedication and professionalism always ensure that our patients receive the best possible care. I am grateful for Dr. Margaret Stolarczuk, who has with great expertise provided outstanding echographic studies of our patients. I am deeply appreciative of the outstanding photography performed by Michael McKenzie and Kimberly Littlefield. Devorah Novak has with perfect accuracy calculated our radiation treatments. Drs. Sarah Huang and John Meyer, with their talents and skill as radiation oncologists and their compassion, have given not only unparalleled care but comfort and trust to our patients.

My good friend, Dr. John Doemeny, provided invaluable assistance for the section on magnetic resonance imaging and authored the explanation of the physics of this technology.

I am indebted to Dr. Edward W. D. Norton and the staff of the Bascom Palmer Eye Institute library, who created an incomparable resource for research and writing.

And finally, I am grateful for Drs. David Abramson, Andrew Schachat, and Karl Olsen, who all carefully read this book and offered their important insight and suggestions.

Malignant melanoma **(Fig. 1.1)** represents a complex pr...
that continues to challenge ophthalmologists. Accurate dia...
sis requires recognition of the potential for many varied clin...
presentations. Some patients with a choroidal or ciliary bo...
malignant melanoma are asymptomatic, while rarely, some have
acute symptoms such as marked inflammation, pain, and loss of

change over many years.
a choroidal or ciliary boc
terns can mimic severa
In large series, th
(AFIP) found that ab
presumed malignan
rently, diagnostic a
occurs in no more
contributed to imp
frequent use of in
of commonly co
domelanomas (T
fluorescein ang
lesions,[77,95,96] an
aspiration biop
always yield
istic features
tests occur.
tic tests, an
a diagnosti
Once
relative a
ment op
plexity
troversi

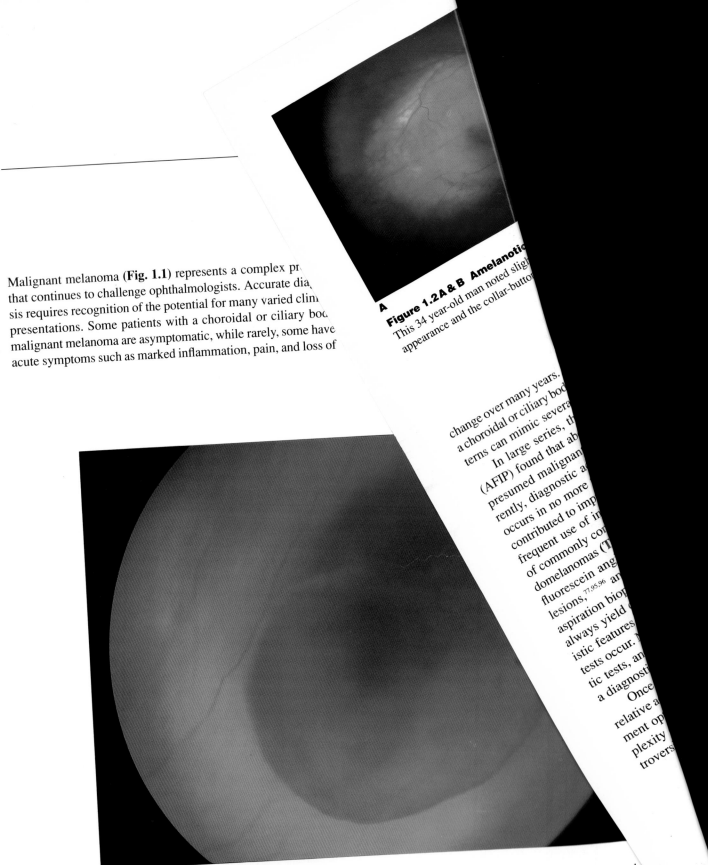

A
Figure 1.2A & B Amelanotic
This 34 year-old man noted slight
appearance and the collar-butto

Figure 1.1 Pigmented Choroidal Malignant Melanoma
This 65 year-old man was found to have a pigmented lesion in his left eye. Visual acuity was 20/30. Note the darkly pigmented r...
collar-button shape. The maximal thickness measured 7.4 mm.

ACKNOWLEDGMENTS

In reflecting over the time this book has been underway, many people have affected this project directly or indirectly and have provided invaluable assistance for which I am extremely grateful.

First of all, I wish to thank my associates, Drs. Howard Schatz and H. Richard McDonald. Their encouragement, support, and extensive knowledge and expertise make our relationship and association beyond compare. I am very grateful for this unique association, which allows me to share both work and friendship with such compassionate and gifted physicians.

I am indebted to Dr. J. Donald M. Gass, whose tremendous insight and gift for observation and understanding made my fellowship with him an exceptional experience. I am deeply appreciative of Drs. Robert Ellsworth and David Abramson, who shared freely with me their extensive experience, insight and knowledge of ocular oncology during my fellowship with them. I am thankful for Drs. George Blankenship, John Clarkson, Harry Flynn, Don Nicholson, and Karl Olsen, who patiently taught me my skills as a vitreoretinal surgeon. John Hungerford allowed me a rewarding opportunity to share in the considerable ocular oncology experience of St. Bartholomew's and Moorfields hospital. May Dr. Alex Irvine never lose the energy, patience and dedication to resident teaching that provided me a unique experience as a resident at the University of California, San Francisco. Dr. Jerry Shields shared his patients and knowledge with me. Dr. Devron Char first stimulated my interest in tumors.

A special thank you to all of the members of and contributors to the Northern California Section of the Collaborative Ocular Melanoma Study. The commitment, time, energy and contributions of these individuals have made ours a busy oncology center. To: Robert T. Wendel, Robert S. Fantl, Edwin E. Boldrey, Donald E. Roy, Stanley Galas, Michael W. Gaynon, W. James Gealy, John H. Drouilhet, Conor C. O'Malley, Roger D. Griffith, Sterling J. Haidt, Steven C. Johnson, Neil E. Kelly, Thomas C. Salzano, James W. Wells, Arthur W. Allen, Jr., Peter F. Petersen, Otto G. Klein, Arnold J. Smoller, Glynne Couvillion, Stephen D. Miller, Michael P. Teske, Gregory S. Brinton, Roy A. Goodart, Everett Ai, Eric J. Del Piero, Geoffrey V. Cecchi, F. Temple Riekhof, Gregory C. Tesluk, Patrick Coonan, Peter R. Egbert, and Greer Geiger.

Karen Laughlin and Anne Miller, the administrators and coordinators of our oncology center, have given so much of themselves to our patients by providing compassionate support, understanding, and a willing ear; their dedication and professionalism always ensure that our patients receive the best possible care. I am grateful for Dr. Margaret Stolarczuk, who has with great expertise provided outstanding echographic studies of our patients. I am deeply appreciative of the outstanding photography performed by Michael McKenzie and Kimberly Littlefield. Devorah Novak has with perfect accuracy calculated our radiation treatments. Drs. Sarah Huang and John Meyer, with their talents and skill as radiation oncologists and their compassion, have given not only unparalleled care but comfort and trust to our patients.

My good friend, Dr. John Doemeny, provided invaluable assistance for the section on magnetic resonance imaging and authored the explanation of the physics of this technology.

I am indebted to Dr. Edward W. D. Norton and the staff of the Bascom Palmer Eye Institute library, who created an incomparable resource for research and writing.

And finally, I am grateful for Drs. David Abramson, Andrew Schachat, and Karl Olsen, who all carefully read this book and offered their important insight and suggestions.

CHAPTER 1

DIAGNOSIS

Malignant melanoma (**Fig. 1.1**) represents a complex problem that continues to challenge ophthalmologists. Accurate diagnosis requires recognition of the potential for many varied clinical presentations. Some patients with a choroidal or ciliary body malignant melanoma are asymptomatic, while rarely, some have acute symptoms such as marked inflammation, pain, and loss of vision. The shape of a melanoma can vary from a well-defined mass to a diffuse tumor that extensively involves the uvea and produces only mild thickening. Some melanomas are deeply pigmented, while others contain no clinically discernible pigmentation (**Fig. 1.2**). Also, the rate of growth differs since some lesions appear to change quickly, while others show little or no

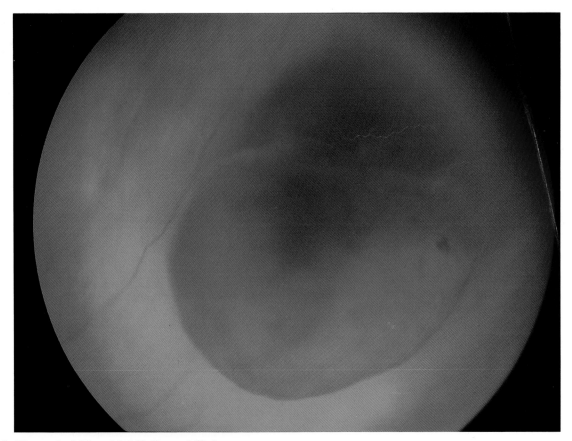

Figure 1.1 Pigmented Choroidal Malignant Melanoma
This 65 year-old man was found to have a pigmented lesion in his left eye. Visual acuity was 20/30. Note the darkly pigmented mass in a collar-button shape. The maximal thickness measured 7.4 mm.

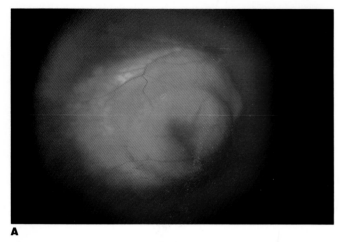
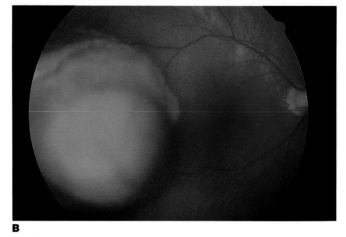

A   B

Figure 1.2 A & B Amelanotic Choroidal Malignant Melanoma
This 34 year-old man noted slight blurring of his vision in his right eye for the past year. The visual acuity was 20/32. Note the amelanotic appearance and the collar-button shape. Standardized echography measured the maximal thickness as 7.1 mm.

change over many years. Although certain features are classic for a choroidal or ciliary body malignant melanoma, these varied patterns can mimic several benign and other malignant disorders.

In large series, the Armed Forces Institute of Pathology (AFIP) found that about 20% of eyes enucleated because of a presumed malignant melanoma were misdiagnosed.[36,80] Currently, diagnostic accuracy is better such that a misdiagnosis occurs in no more than 3% of eyes.[2,21,31,76] Several factors have contributed to improved accuracy in diagnosis, including more frequent use of indirect ophthalmoscopy, enhanced awareness of commonly confused lesions that are sometimes called pseudomelanomas (**Table 1.1**), development of ultrasonography and fluorescein angiography, judicious observation of suspicious lesions,[77,95,96] and most recently, the application of fine needle aspiration biopsy.[9,10,21,24,28,30,47] These diagnostic modalities do not always yield definitive diagnoses, and exceptions to characteristic features of malignant melanoma ascribed to each of these tests occur. Nevertheless, reliance on a combination of diagnostic tests, and an understanding of their limitations, can achieve a diagnostic accuracy of about 99%.[19,21,26,57,72,77]

Once a diagnosis of malignant melanoma is established, the relative advantages and disadvantages of several potential treatment options must be considered. Adding further to the complexity of this subject are widely divergent opinions and controversies regarding diagnosis and treatment.[19,21,42,48,62,74,76]

Table 1.1
Pseudomelanomas

Choroidal Nevus	Combined Retinal-RPE[†]
Macular Disciform Scar	Hamartoma
Eccentric Disciform Scar	Luxated Lens
CHRPE[*]	Cavernous Hemangioma of the
Choroidal Hemangioma	Retina
Reactive RPE[†] Hyperplasia	Central Retinal Vein
Melanocytoma	Obstruction
Choroidal Detachment	Reticulum Cell Sarcoma
Hemorrhagic RPE[†] or Retinal	Toxoplasmosis
Detachment	Macular Pucker
Vitreous Hemorrhage	Subretinal Granuloma
Rhegmatogenous Retinal	Histoplasmosis
Detachment	RPE[†] or Ciliary Epithelial
Posterior Scleritis	Adenoma
Metastatic Carcinoma	Myopic Chorioretinal
Retinoschisis	Degeneration
Uveal Effusion Syndrome	Retinitis, Viral
Choroidal Osteoma	

[*] CHRPE—Congenital Hypertrophy of Retinal Pigment Epithelium
[†] RPE—Retinal Pigment Epithelial
(Adapted from Shields, JA, Augsburger, JJ, Brown, GC, Stephens, RF: The differential diagnosis of posterior uveal melanoma. Ophthalmology 87:518-522, 1980.)

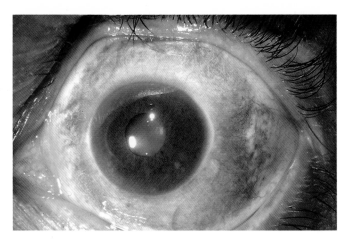

Figure 1.3 Melanosis Oculi
This 67 year-old female with melanosis oculi was diagnosed with a large malignant melanoma in this eye. Note the increased episclera pigmentation.

cases have occurred, but this also is unusual.[18,34] Racial risk factors are well recognized. Data from the Third National Cancer Survey in the United States suggest that malignant melanoma is eight times more frequent in whites than in nonwhites.[68]

Two congenital conditions, melanosis oculi (**Fig. 1.3**) and nevus of Ota,[34,37,44,87,93] are a risk factor for the development of malignant melanoma, though some believe that the frequency of this association is overestimated.[13] Both melanosis oculi and nevus of Ota are conditions in which there is unilateral hyperpigmentation of the episclera and uveal tract. In addition, nevus of Ota (oculodermal melanocytosis) has associated ipsilateral hyperpigmentation of the periorbital skin. Nevus of Ota is more common in blacks and Asians, but malignant transformation is more common in whites. Approximately 5% of patients with nevus of Ota will have bilateral involvement. Some case reports of uveal malignant melanoma occurring in patients with the familial atypical multiple mole melanoma syndrome (dysplastic nevus syndrome, B-K mole syndrome, **Fig. 1.4**) suggest there may be an increased risk in patients with this syndrome,[1,67] but controversy exists concerning this association.[34,45,83]

EPIDEMIOLOGICAL FEATURES

Malignant melanoma is the most common primary ocular malignancy and each year approximately six to seven cases of malignant melanoma per million people are diagnosed in the United States (approximately 1,500 cases).[12,48,68,89] The median age at the time of diagnosis is about 55 years,[48,61] and occurrence under age 20 is rare.[6,11,12,27,34,48] There is a similar risk for both sexes.[48,68,84] Bilateral occurrence is very rare[52,69,70] and is estimated to occur in the United States only once every 18 years.[70] A few familial

MEDICAL AND OCULAR HISTORY

A careful history is extremely important. Information should be sought that can assist in forming a differential diagnosis. A review of symptoms may reveal a prior mastectomy or elicit pulmonary or gastrointestinal symptoms that suggest a primary

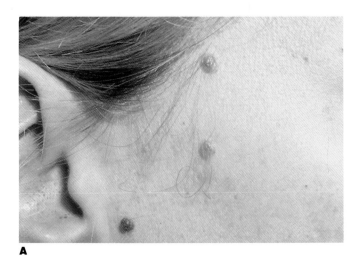

A

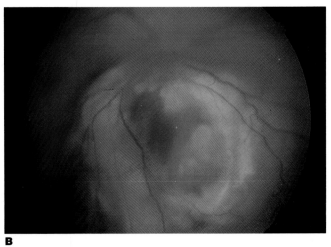

B

Figure 1.4 A & B Dysplastic Nevus Syndrome and Choroidal Malignant Melanoma
This 37 year-old female has B-K mole syndrome (dysplastic nevus syndrome, Figure 1.4A). She had a history of skin melanoma and was also found to have a choroidal malignant melanoma (Figure 1.4B). Note the amelanotic malignant melanoma with overlying hemorrhage.

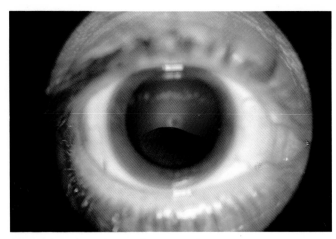

Figure 1.5 Anterior Malignant Melanoma
This 48 year-old female noted a superior shadow and blurred vision for approximately 3 weeks. A large ciliary body and anterior choroidal mass was present. A dark tumor can be seen in the lower portion of the pupil. The basal diameter of this mass was 13 mm × 13 mm and the maximal height by standardized echography was 12.6 mm.

malignancy in these organs. Such a history necessitates consideration of metastatic eye disease as the cause of an ocular mass lesion.[72,82] Prior trauma may suggest a retinal pigment epithelial proliferation as an unusual cause of a pigmented mass.[85] Additionally, recent ocular surgery should suggest postoperative choroidal detachment associated with hypotony.[72]

Symptoms

Most patients with a malignant melanoma are symptomatic, and historically, about 5% of patients were asymptomatic.[48,97] More recently, with increased use of indirect ophthalmoscopy, more patients are found to have a melanoma during a routine examination.[20]

Patients may experience photopsias, blurred vision, metamorphopsia, and visual field changes.[21,29,62,72,74] A ciliary body melanoma (**Fig. 1.5**) may enlarge toward the lens and produce astigmatism, cataract, or subluxation.[29,74] A posterior choroidal melanoma may directly involve the fovea or leak fluid under the retina (**Fig. 1.6**). When a small amount of subretinal fluid affects

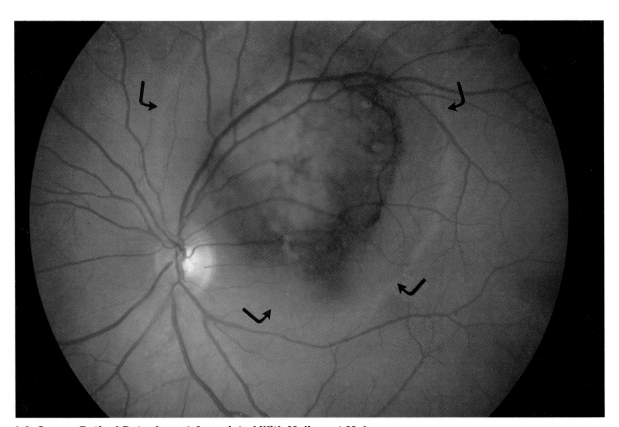

Figure 1.6 Serous Retinal Detachment Associated With Malignant Melanoma
This 32 year-old female noted blurred vision in her left eye for approximately 2 years. Best corrected visual acuity was 20/80. A pigmented lesion extends superiorly from the macula. There is a shallow overlying serous retinal detachment (arrows) that extends into the fovea. Orange lipofuscin pigment is present over the surface of the tumor.

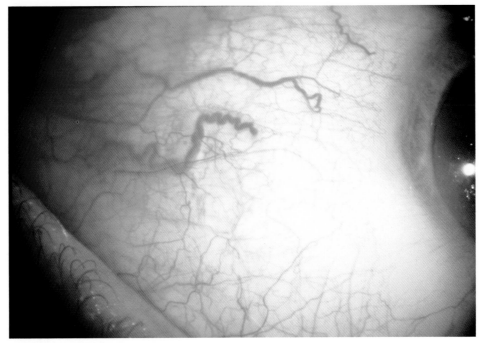

Figure 1.7 Sentinel Vessels
Note the dilated episcleral vessels (sentinel vessels) that were present over a large anterior choroidal malignant melanoma.

the fovea, a patient can notice metamorphopsia and blurred vision. Other patients may have good central vision but note a reduced visual field caused by peripheral retinal detachment. In contrast, a patient with prior poor vision in an eye may not recognize some of these earlier changes since they may only produce mild visual symptoms. Patients unaware of a problem will not seek help, and the diagnosis will be delayed.[5]

Occasionally, a change in the external appearance of the eye draws attention to it. Dilated episcleral vessels overlying the area of a tumor (so-called sentinel vessels, **Fig. 1.7**) can cause a red eye. Or, intraocular inflammation can cause conjunctival congestion and a red eye.[21,29,41,48,62] Infrequently, an area of increased bulbar pigmentation may be observed by some patients; this is only occasionally caused by extraocular tumor extension.

Pain is unusual except with large tumors that have caused glaucoma, necrosis and inflammation, or extraocular extension.[21,62,74] In the past, ocular inflammation occurred as an early sign of malignant melanoma in roughly 5% of cases,[41] but it is probably an even less frequent presenting symptom of malignant melanoma today.

OCULAR EXAMINATION

Slit-Lamp Examination and Intraocular Pressure

Slit-lamp examination may show epibulbar pigmentation or dilated, engorged episcleral vessels overlying the tumor. Anterior uveitis is observed in up to 21% of cases.[48,51,61] A ciliary body melanoma may be clearly visible through a dilated pupil (**Fig. 1.5**), and in some ciliary body melanomas, gonioscopic examination may prove invasion of the angle structures.

In a recent series, 2% of eyes with a choroidal melanoma and 17% of eyes with a ciliary body melanoma had an increased intraocular pressure.[71] Etiologies for increased intraocular pressure include angle closure caused by rubeosis, inflammation, or anterior displacement of the iris-lens diaphragm.[61,62,71,91] Glaucoma is more frequent in eyes with larger or more anterior melanomas or when a total retinal detachment is present.[15,48,62,91] Infrequently, pigment-laden macrophages and melanoma cells may disperse within the anterior chamber or vitreous. This is most commonly associated with tumor necrosis and ciliary body melanomas. Accumulation in the anterior chamber may produce a black hypopyon.[4] Alternatively, these cells can obstruct the trabecular meshwork and produce what has been called "melanomalytic glaucoma."[35,56,71,86,92]

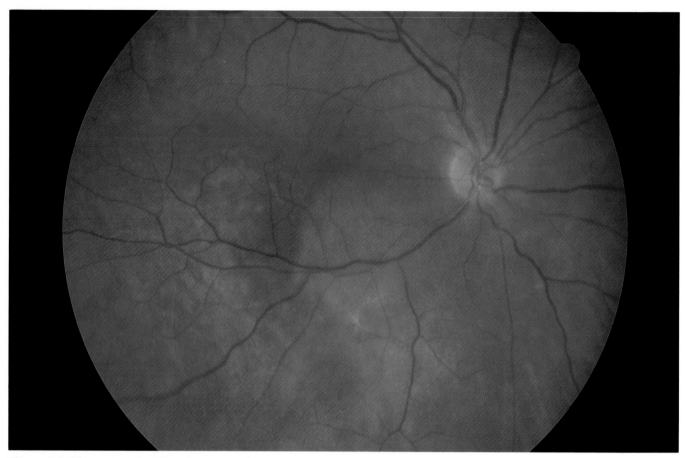

Figure 1.8 Pigmented And Nonpigmented Choroidal Malignant Melanoma
This 53 year-old female was diagnosed with a medium-sized malignant melanoma. Areas of the tumor are pigmented while other areas are amelanotic.

Indirect Ophthalmoscopy

With clear ocular media, indirect ophthalmoscopy is often diagnostic.[19,21,42,48,62,74,76] A careful examination of the fellow eye is essential since clues to the correct diagnosis, such as the presence of other masses or macular degeneration, may be obtained.[62,72] Most malignant melanomas have a grayish-brown color (**Fig. 1.1**), but approximately 20% to 25% appear yellowish-white (amelanotic, **Fig. 1.2**). Sometimes, portions of the tumor may be amelanotic while adjacent areas are deeply pigmented (**Fig. 1.8**). The shape may be discoid or like a dome (**Fig. 1.9A**) or a collar-button

(**Fig. 1.9B**). The latter appearance occurs when a portion of the melanoma has squeezed through a disruption in Bruch's membrane. There is less resistance to growth within the subretinal space compared with the choroid and this allows the extruded portion of the melanoma to enlarge. Growth may appear rapid (**Fig. 1.9**), but this is probably due to loss of the restraining effect of Bruch's membrane and not due to increased mitotic activity. A collar-button shape is virtually pathognomonic for a choroidal melanoma since other choroidal tumors, such as metastatic masses or hemangiomas, rarely develop this appearance.[19,21] One unusual manifestation of a collar-button is the presence of

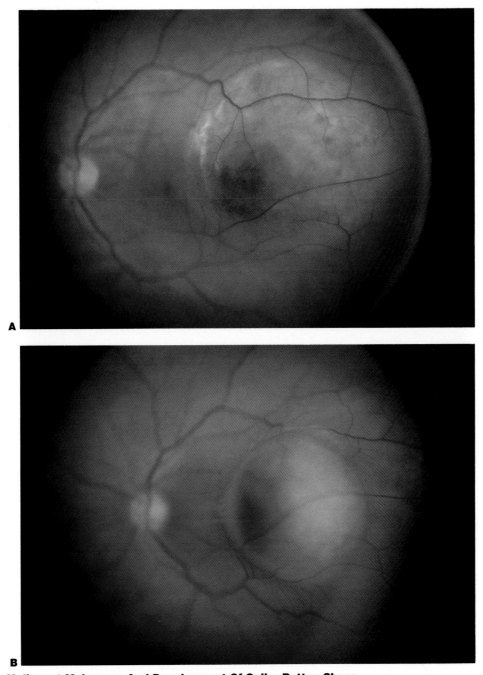

Figure 1.9 A & B Malignant Melanoma And Development Of Collar-Button Shape
This 31 year-old male was found to have reduced vision 3 weeks earlier during an eye exam at the Department of Motor Vehicles. Best corrected vision was 20/50. Note the pigmented tumor involving the fovea and extending temporally (Figure 1.9A). The maximal height was measured as 5.7 mm. Three weeks later (Figure 1.9B), a collar-button configuration developed and the maximal height was now 7.4 mm.

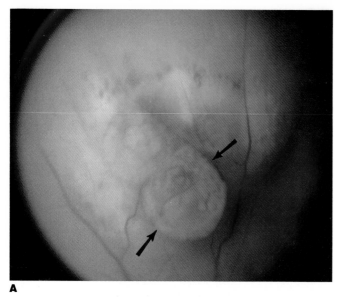

A

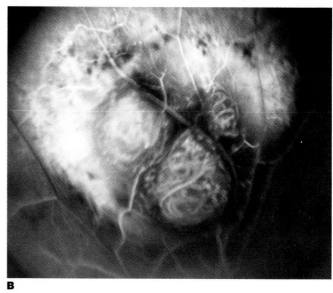

B

Figure 1.10A & B Prominent Vascularity Of Collar-Button Lesion
This 63 year-old man was found to have this amelanotic tumor during a routine examination. There was an unusual appearance of 3 small collar-buttons over the surface of the lesion (Figure 1.10A, arrow). There was prominent vascularity present within one of the collar-button-shaped protrusions. This vascularity was very apparent on a fluorescein angiogram (Figure 1.10B).

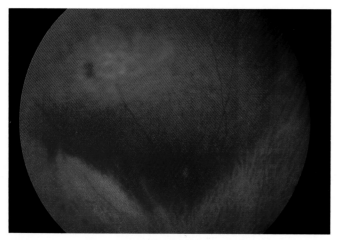

Figure 1.11 Diffuse Choroidal Malignant Melanoma
A 72 year-old male had reduced vision of 20/80 in his left eye and a diffuse malignant melanoma. Maximal thickness was 2.6 mm.

markedly dilated vessels within the tumor apex **(Fig. 1.10)**, which appears similar to an angioma.[42,49,84,90] Strangulation by Bruch's membrane, and subsequent congestion of blood vessels within the protruding portion is cited as a probable cause but only rarely does this produce vitreous hemorrhage.[48,62]

Instead of a discrete tumor mass, a diffuse pattern of growth, involving one-quarter or more of the fundus, occurs in approximately 5% of cases **(Fig. 1.11)**.[40,63,94] This growth pattern typically produces a mild choroidal thickening of only 3 mm to 5 mm and may make the diagnosis difficult.[40,48] Generally, a diffuse melanoma has a poorer prognosis for survival.

A ciliary body tumor may extend within the ciliary body around the globe and is called a ring melanoma.[54,62] Rarely, a ciliary body melanoma may have a multicentric origin.[22]

A full evaluation of an intraocular mass requires estimating its basal diameter and height. Although skilled ultrasonography is the most accurate method for measuring apical height, it is less useful for estimating basal diameters. This is because the sloping margins of a mass are frequently not elevated enough to permit exact determination of the tumor border. Indirect ophthalmoscopy or slit-lamp biomicroscopy is more useful to determine the diameter. Frequently, tumor dimensions are compared with the disc (generally considered to be 1.5 mm in diameter).

Various alterations may be observed ophthalmoscopically over the surface of a malignant melanoma, such as areas of reti-

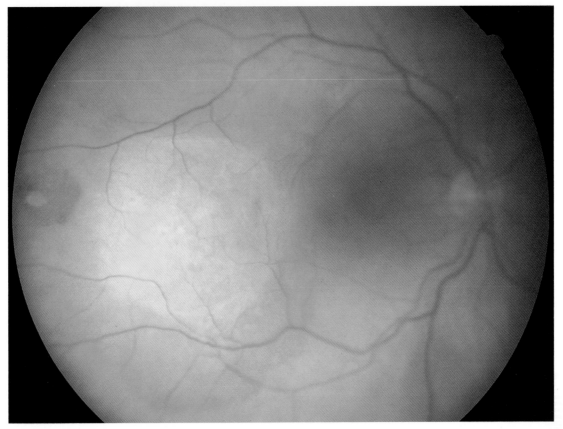

Figure 1.12 Orange Lipofuscin Pigment

This 78 year-old female noted the recent onset of blurred vision in her right eye. The best corrected visual acuity was 20/70. A pigmented tumor was present temporal to the fovea. Orange lipofuscin pigment can be seen over the surface of the mass. The maximal thickness was 3.9 mm.

nal pigment epithelial proliferation, drusen formation, and orange pigment clumps.[21,72,79,81,88] These orange pigment clumps **(Fig. 1.12)** are accumulations of lipofuscin within macrophages presumably produced by degeneration of the retinal pigment epithelium overlying the melanoma. Although these clumps occur occasionally over nevi,[21] their presence is more consistent with a malignant melanoma[81] and suggest an increased probability of future tumor growth.[43] Lipofuscin overlying pigmented tumors often looks orangish, whereas it appears light or medium brown when overlying an amelanotic malignant melanoma and reddish or dull brown over metastatic lesions.[79] This variability of the color results from alterations in the contrast and illumination produced by different colored tumors. Pigment-laden macrophages or melanoma cells dispersed within the vitreous may settle and produce preretinal foci. A bone-spiculated pattern of these settled cells may give a pseudoretinitis pigmentosa appearance.[33] A yellowish halo may be visible surrounding the base of some melanomas due to large pale cells that are sometimes present along the periphery of a malignant melanoma and are called balloon cells **(Fig. 1.13)**.

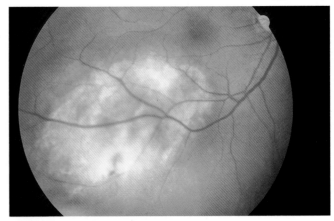

Figure 1.13 Balloon Cells and Malignant Choroidal Melanoma

This 41 year-old female noted a blind spot in her right eye for 6 weeks. Visual acuity was 20/20. The maximal thickness of this malignant melanoma was 3.7 mm. Note the unusual yellowish halo that was most prominent nasally due to the presence of balloon cells. (Photo courtesy of David Abramson, MD).

Subretinal fluid **(Fig. 1.14)** is frequently present,[8,48] though the retina usually remains attached over the apex of the tumor unless there is extensive retinal detachment.[62] A total retinal detachment is particularly common with large or diffuse tumors.[64] Classically, the borders of an exudative retinal detachment will shift with a change in the position of the patient's head. Shifting fluid is common with secondary retinal detachments but unusual with rhegmatogenous retinal detachments.[16,72] Subretinal hemorrhage **(Fig. 1.15)** occurs in about 20% of eyes,[8] a condition generally associated with larger lesions and Bruch's membrane rupture.[21] Up to 5% of patients with a choroidal melanoma will have a vitreous hemorrhage.[8,41]

Tumor necrosis, particularly when extensive, can alter the clinical appearance and make the diagnosis more difficult.[14,17,23,63,64] Establishing the correct diagnosis of a necrotic melanoma also may be difficult because the ultrasonographic features typical of a malignant melanoma may be altered.[23,62] Two clinical presentations of a necrotic tumor, each associated with a distinct histopathologic appearance have been described.[63] One type usually produces blurred vision, and less frequently, pain. Clinically, inflammation is always present, and "choroiditis" is the most frequent initial diagnosis. Most often, a long delay precedes the correct diagnosis. The second clinical presentation of tumor necrosis also often has a history of inflammation (uveitis or scleritis). However, the inflammation worsens abruptly heralded by a sudden onset of pain and blurred vision. The correct diagnosis can usually be made with less delay in these cases because of the sudden increase in symptoms and signs. Less commonly, this latter type can mimic panophthalmitis because of marked inflammation, pain, swollen eyelids and conjunctiva **(Fig. 1.16)**.[60]

The Eye With Opaque Media

Any eye with opaque media should be suspected to have a malignant melanoma.[19,21,23,42,48,62,74,76] The causes of opaque media in eyes

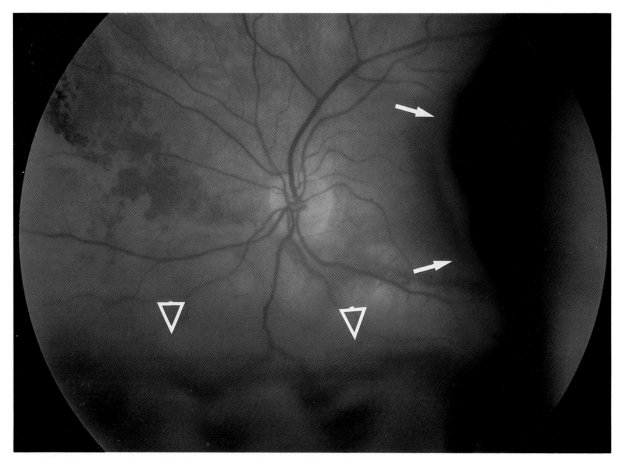

Figure 1.14 Malignant Choroidal Melanoma With Exudative Retinal Detachment
This 71 year-old female noted progressive loss of peripheral vision for one week. Visual acuity was 20/25. A large temporal malignant melanoma (arrows) was present that extended to the ora serrata and measured 8.4 mm thick. An inferior exudative retinal detachment is present that appears dark because of substantial subretinal hemorrhage (arrowheads).

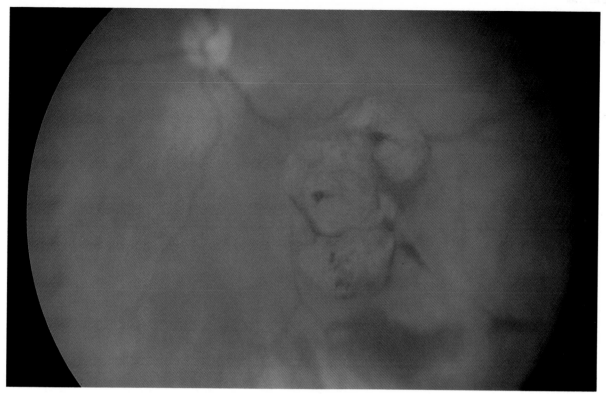

Figure 1.15 Subretinal Hemorrhage and Malignant Choroidal Melanoma
This 67 year-old female noted blurred vision in her left eye for several months. The best corrected visual acuity was 20/40. Note the pigmented tumor inferior to the macula that has a triple collar-button configuration. Subretinal hemorrhage is present along the inferior border of an overlying retinal detachment.

that contain a malignant melanoma include corneal edema, hyphema, cataract and vitreous hemorrhage.[74,78] Some reports have indicated that as many as 22% of enucleated eyes with melanoma have opaque media.[36,53,78,80,95] More recent experience indicates that this number is decreasing, probably because a diagnosis of malignant melanoma is being made earlier.[97]

The diagnosis of malignant melanoma in eyes with opaque media may be difficult.[23,59,62,78] Careful ultrasonographic evaluation should be done to search for a possible malignant melanoma. Eyes with opaque cataracts should have a preoperative examination that includes B-scan ultrasonography besides A-scan intraocular lens measurements.[25,59,75] This may be particularly important in eyes with asymmetric lenticular opacities.

Most commonly, patients with a malignant melanoma are symptomatic and have blurred or altered vision. Improved awareness of the differential diagnosis of intraocular masses and more frequent use of indirect ophthalmoscopy, fluorescein angiography, and ultrasonography, has substantially improved detection of an intraocular mass and diagnostic accuracy. Less common presentations do occur, but a high degree of suspicion and additional diagnostic studies can usually provide the correct answer.

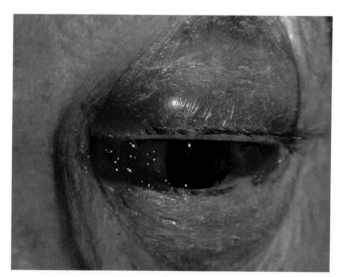

Figure 1.16 Necrotic Malignant Choroidal Melanoma Presenting As Panophthalmitis
This 52 year-old man was previously told that he had a small melanoma. Sixteen months later, he presented with a 4 day history of severe ocular redness and pain. Examination demonstrated a blind left eye, periorbital swelling, proptosis, and hemorrhagic chemosis. Enucleation was done, and a necrotic melanoma confirmed.

REFERENCES

1. Abramson DH, Rodriquez-Sains RS, Rubman R: B-K mole syndrome. Cutaneous and ocular malignant melanoma. Arch Ophthalmol 98:1397-1399, 1980.

2. Addison DJ, Wakelin DL: Errors in the diagnosis of choroidal malignant melanoma. Can J Ophthalmol 10:205-206, 1975.

3. Albert, D: Toward resolving the ocular melanoma controversy. Arch Ophthalmol 97:451-452, 1979.

4. Albert DM, Lahav M, Torczynski E, et al.: Black hypopyon: Report of two cases. Graefes Arch Clin Exp Ophthalmol 193:81-93, 1975.

5. Albert DM, Zakov ZN, Smith TR: Late diagnosis of choroidal malignant melanomas in eyes with clear media and low visual acuity. Trans Am Acad Ophthalmol 86:1037-1047, 1979.

6. Apt L: Uveal melanomas in children and adolescents. Int Ophthalmol Clinic 2:403-410, 1962.

7. Augsburger JJ: Does treatment improve or worsen the survival rate of patients? Ophthalmology (supp) 95:147, 1988.

8. Augsburger JJ, Golden MI, Shields JA: Fluorescein angiography of choroidal malignant melanomas with retinal invasion. Retina 4:232-241, 1984.

9. Augsburger JJ, Shields JA: Fine needle aspiration biopsy of solid intraocular tumors: indications, instrumentation and techniques. Ophthalmic Surg 15:34-40, 1984.

10. Augsburger JJ, Shields JA, Folberg R, et al.: Fine needle aspiration biopsy in the diagnosis of intraocular cancer. Cytologic-histologic correlations. Ophthalmology 92:39-49, 1985.

11. Barr CC, McLean IW, Zimmerman LE: Uveal melanoma in children and adolescents. Arch Ophthalmol 99:2133-2136, 1981.

12. Birdsell JM, Gunther BK, Boyd TA, et al.: Ocular melanoma: A population-based study. Can J Ophthalmol 15:9-12, 1980.

13. Blodi FC: Ocular melanocytosis and melanoma. Am J Ophthalmol 80:389-395, 1975.

14. Blodi FC: Pathology of choroidal melanomas. Unusual aspects confusing the clinical diagnosis. Trans Ophthalmol Soc UK 97:362-367, 1977.

15. Boniuk M: A crisis in the management of patients with choroidal melanoma. Editorial. Am J Ophthalmol 87:840-841, 1979.

16. Boniuk M, Zimmerman LE: Occurrence and behavior of choroidal melanomas in eyes subjected to operations for retinal detachment. Tr Amer Acad Ophthalmol Oto 66:642-658, 1962.

17. Bujara K: Necrotic malignant melanomas of the choroid and ciliary body. A clinicopathological and statistical study. Albrecht von Graefes Arch Klin Exp Ophthalmol 219:40-43, 1982.

18. Canning CR, Hungerford J: Familial uveal melanoma. Br J Ophthalmol 72:241-243, 1988.

19. Char DH: The management of small choroidal melanomas. Surv Ophthalmol 22:377-386, 1978.

20. Char DH: Therapeutic options in uveal melanoma. Editorial. Am J Ophthalmol 98:796-799, 1984.

21. Char DH: Clinical Ocular Oncology. New York, Churchill Livingstone, 1989, pp 91-149.

22. Char DH, Crawford JB, Gonzales J, Miller T: Iris melanoma with increased intraocular pressure. Differentiation of focal solitary tumors from diffuse or multiple tumors. Arch Ophthalmol 107:548-551, 1989.

23. Char DH, Howes EL, Fries PD, et al.: Uveal melanoma with opaque media: Absence of definitive diagnosis before enucleation. Can J Ophthalmol 23:22-26, 1988.

24. Char DH, Miller TR, Ljung BM, et al.: Fine needle aspiration biopsy in uveal melanoma. Presented at Advances and Controversies in the Management of Ocular and Periocular Malignancies. San Francisco, December, 1988.

25. Chess J, Henkind P, Albert DM, et al.: Uveal melanoma presenting after cataract extraction with intraocular lens implantation. Ophthalmology 92:827-830, 1985.

26. Collaborative Ocular Melanoma Study Group: Accuracy of diagnosis of choroidal melanomas in the Collaborative Ocular Melanoma Study. Arch Ophthalmol 108: 1268-1273, 1990.

27. Cury D, Lucie H, Irvine AR: Prepubertal intraocular malignant melanoma. Am J Ophthalmol 47(5) pp 2:202-206, 1959.

28. Czerniak B, Woyke S, Domagala W, Krzysztolik Z: Fine needle aspiration cytology of intraocular malignant melanoma. Acta Cytologica 27:157-165, 1983.

29. Damato BE, Foulds WS: Ciliary body tumours and their management. Tr Ophthalmol Soc UK 105:257-264, 1986.

30. Davey CC, Deery ARS: Through the eye, a needle: Intraocular fine needle aspiration biopsy. Tr Ophthalmol Soc UK 105:78-83, 1986.

31. Davidorf FH, Letson AD, Weiss ET, Levine E: Incidence of misdiagnosed and unsuspected choroidal melanomas. A 50-year experience. Arch Ophthalmol 101:410-412, 1983.

32. Davidorf FH, McAdoo JF: Enucleation for choroidal melanoma. In Schachat, AP (Ed): Retina. St. Louis, CV Mosby, 1989, vol. 1, pp 687-691.

33. Eagle R, Shields JA: Pseudoretinitis pigmentosa secondary to preretinal malignant melanoma cells. Retina 2:51-55, 1982.

34. Egan KM, Seddon JM, Glynn RJ, et al.: Epidemiologic aspects of uveal melanoma. Surv Ophthalmol 32:239-251, 1988.

35. El Baba F, Hagler WS, De La Cruz A, Green WR: Choroidal melanoma with pigment dispersion in vitreous and melanomalytic glaucoma. Ophthalmology 95:370-377, 1988.

36. Ferry AP: Lesions mistaken for malignant melanoma of the posterior uvea. Arch Ophthalmol 72:463-469, 1964.

37. Ferry AP: Congenital melanosis oculi and its relationship to uveal malignant melanoma. In Lommatzsch PK, Blodi FC (Eds): Intraocular Tumors. New York, Springer-Verlag, 1983, pp 58-65.

38. Fine SL: Do I take the eye out or leave it in? Arch Ophthalmol 104:653-654, 1986.

39. Fine SL: Controversy in the management of choroidal and ciliary body melanoma. Ophthalmology (Suppl) 95:147, 1988.

40. Font RL, Spaulding AG, Zimmerman LE: Diffuse malignant melanoma of the uveal tract: A clinicopathologic report of 54 cases. Tr Amer Acad Ophthalmol Oto 72:877-894, 1968.

41. Fraser DJ, Font RL: Ocular inflammation and hemorrhage as initial manifestations of uveal malignant melanoma. Arch Ophthalmol 97:1311-1314, 1979.

42. Gass JDM: Fluorescein angiography. An aid in the differential diagnosis of intraocular tumors. Int Ophthalmol Clin 12:85-120, 1972.

43. Gass JDM: Observation of suspected choroidal and ciliary body melanomas for evidence of growth prior to enucleation. Ophthalmology 87:523-528, 1980.

44. Gonder JR, Shields JA, Albert DM, et al.: Uveal malignant melanoma associated with ocular and oculodermal melanocytosis. Ophthalmology 89:953-960, 1982.

45. Greene MH, Sanders RJ, Chu FC, et al.: The familial occurrence of cutaneous melanoma, intraocular melanoma, and the dysplastic nevus syndrome. Am J Ophthalmol 96:238-245, 1983.

46. Jakobiec FA: A moratorium on enucleation for choroidal melanoma? Editorial. Am J Ophthalmol 87:842-846, 1979.

47. Jakobiec FA, Coleman DJ, Chattock A, Smith M: Ultrasonically guided needle biopsy and cytologic diagnosis of solid intraocular tumors. Tr Am Acad Ophthalmol Oto 86:1662-1681, 1979.

48. Jensen OA: Malignant melanomas of the uvea in Denmark 1943-1952. A clinical, histopathological, and prognostic study. Acta Ophthalmol (Suppl) 75:1-220, 1963.

49. Jensen OA: The "Knapp-Ronne" type of malignant melanoma of the choroid. A haemangioma-like melanoma with a typical clinical picture. Acta Ophthalmol 54:41-54, 1976.

50. Khalil MK: Balloon cell malignant melanoma of the choroid: Ultrastructural studies. Br J Ophthalmol 67:579-584, 1983.

51. Kirk HO, Petty RW: Malignant melanoma of the choroid. A correlation of clinical and histological findings. Arch Ophthalmol 56:843-860, 1956.

52. Lubin JR, Gragoodas ES, Albert DM, Weichselbaum RR: Bilateral malignant choroidal melanomas. Int Ophthalmol Clin 20:103-115, 1980.

53. Makley TA, Havener WH, Newberg J: Light coagulation of intraocular tumors. Am J Ophthalmol 60:1082-1089, 1965.

54. Manschot WA: Ring melanoma. Arch Ophthalmol 71:625-632, 1964.

55. Maumenee AE: An evaluation of enucleation in the management of uveal melanomas. Editorial. Am J Ophthalmol 87:846-847, 1979.

56. McMenamin PG, Lee WR: Ultrastructural pathology of melanomalytic glaucoma. Br J Ophthalmol 70:895-906, 1986.

57. Oosterhuis JA, De Wolf-Rouendaal D: Differential diagnosis of very small melanomas and naevi of the choroid. In Oosterhuis JA (Ed): Ophthalmic Tumors. Boston, Junk Publishers, 1985, pp 1-8.

58. Packer S: The management of choroidal melanoma. Arch Ophthalmol 102:1450-1451, 1984.

59. Pe'er J, Savino DF, McLean IW, Zimmerman LE: Posterior uveal melanomas in aphakic and pseudophakic eyes. Am J Ophthalmol 101:458-460, 1986.

60. Pizzuto D, deLuise V, Zimmerman N: Choroidal malignant melanoma appearing as acute panophthalmitis. Letter to the Editor. Am J Ophthalmol 101:249-251, 1986.

61. Raivio I: Uveal melanoma in Finland. An epidemiological, clinical, histological and prognostic study. Acta Ophthalmol 133:5-64, 1977.

62. Reese AB: Pigmented tumors. In Tumors of the Eye. Third Ed, New York, Harper & Row, 1976, pp 173-226.

63. Reese AB, Archila EA, Jones IS, Cooper WC: Necrosis of malignant melanomas of the choroid. Am J Ophthalmol 99:104, 1970.

64. Reese AB, Howard GM: Flat uveal melanomas. Am J Ophthalmol 64:1021-1028, 1967.

65. Riley FC: Balloon cell melanoma of the choroid. Arch Ophthalmol 92:131-133, 1974.

66. Rodrigues MM, Shields JA: Malignant melanoma of the choroid with balloon cells. A clinicopathologic study of three cases. Can J Ophthalmol 11:208-215, 1976.

67. Rodriguez-Sains RS: Ocular findings in patients with dysplastic nevus syndrome. Ophthalmology 93:661-665, 1986.

68. Scotto J, Fraumeni JF, Lee JAH: Melanomas of the eye and other noncutaneous sites: Epidemiologic aspects. J Natl Canc Inst 56:489-491, 1976.

69. Seregard S, Daunius C, Kock E, Popovic V: Two cases of primary bilateral malignant melanoma of the choroid. Br J Ophthalmol 72:244-245, 1988.

70. Shammas HF, Watzke RC: Bilateral choroidal melanomas. Case report and incidence. Arch Ophthalmol 95:617-623, 1977.

71. Shields CL, Shields JA, Shields B, Augsburger JJ: Prevalence and mechanisms of secondary intraocular pressure elevation in eyes with intraocular tumors. Ophthalmology 94:839-846, 1987.

72. Shields JA: Current approaches to the diagnosis and management of choroidal melanomas. Surv Ophthalmol 21:443-463, 1977.

73. Shields JA: Counseling the patient with a posterior uveal melanoma. Am J Ophthalmol 106:88-91, 1988.

74. Shields JA: Diagnosis and Management of Intraocular Tumors. St. Louis, CV Mosby 1983.

75. Shields JA, Augsburger JJ: Cataract surgery and intraocular lenses in patients with unsuspected malignant melanoma of the ciliary body and choroid. Ophthalmology 92:823-826, 1985.

76. Shields JA, Augsburger JJ, Brown GC, Stephens RF: The differential diagnosis of posterior uveal melanoma. Ophthalmology 87:518-522, 1980.

77. Shields JA, McDonald PR: Improvements in the diagnosis of posterior uveal melanomas. Arch Ophthalmol 91:259-264, 1974.

78. Shields JA, McDonald PR, Leonard BC, Canny CLB: The diagnosis of uveal malignant melanomas in eyes with opaque media. Am J Ophthalmol 83:95-105, 1977.

79. Shields JA, Rodrigues MM, Sarin LK, et al.: Lipofuscin pigment over benign and malignant choroidal tumors. Trans Am Acad Ophthalmol Oto 81:871-881, 1976.

80. Shields JA, Zimmerman LE: Lesions simulating malignant melanoma of the posterior uvea. Arch Ophthalmol 89:466-471, 1973.

81. Smith LT, Irvine AR: Diagnostic significance of orange pigment accumulation over choroidal tumors. Am J Ophthalmol 76:212-216, 1973.

82. Stephens RF, Shields JA: Diagnosis and management of cancer metastatic to the uvea: a study of 70 cases. Ophthalmology 86:1336-1349, 1979.

83. Taylor MR, Guerry D, Bondi EE, et al.: Lack of association between intraocular melanoma and cutaneous dysplastic nevi. Am J Ophthalmol 98:478-482, 1984.

84. Terry TL, Johns JP: Uveal sarcoma-malignant melanoma. A statistical study of ninety-four cases. Am J Ophthalmol 18:903-913, 1935.

85. Tso MOM, Albert DM: Pathological condition of the retinal pigment epithelium. Neoplasms and nodular non-neoplastic lesions. Arch Ophthalmol 88:27-38, 1972.

86. Van Buskirk E, Leure-du Pree, AE: Pathophysiology and electron microscopy of melanomalytic glaucoma. Am J Ophthalmol 85:160-166, 1978.

87. Velazquez N, Jones IS: Ocular and oculodermal melanocytosis associated with uveal melanoma. Ophthalmology 90:1472-1476, 1983.

88. Wallow IHL, Tso MOM: Proliferation of the retinal pigment epithelium over malignant choroidal tumors. A light and electron microscopic study. Am J Ophthalmol 73:914-926, 1972.

89. Wilkes SR, Robertson DM, Kurland LT, Campbell RJ: Incidence of uveal malignant melanoma in the resident population of Rochester and Olmsted county, Minnesota. Am J Ophthalmol 87:639-641, 1979.

90. Wolter JR, Schut AL, Martonyi CL: Hemangioma-like clinical appearance of a collar-button melanoma caused by the strangulation effect of Bruch's membrane. Am J Ophthalmol 76:730-733, 1973.

91. Yanoff M: Glaucoma mechanisms in ocular malignant melanomas. Am J Ophthalmol 70:898-904, 1970.

92. Yanoff M, Scheie HG: Melanomalytic glaucoma. Report of a case. Arch Ophthalmol 84:471-473, 1970.

93. Yanoff M, Zimmerman LE: Histogenesis of malignant melanomas of the uvea. III. The relationship of congenital ocular melanocytosis and neurofibromatosis to uveal melanomas. Arch Ophthalmol 77:331-336, 1967.

94. Zeeman WPC: The diagnosis of the flat sarcoma of the choroid and the histologica substratum of the changes observed with the ophthalmoscope. Acta Ophthalmol 21:47-60, 1944.

95. Zimmerman LE: Problems in the diagnosis of malignant melanomas of the choroid and ciliary body. The 1972 Arthur J. Bedell Lecture. Am J Ophthalmol 75:917-929, 1973.

96. Zimmerman LE, McLean IW: Changing concepts of the prognosis and management of small malignant melanomas of the choroid. Montgomery Lecture, 1975. Tr Ophthalmol Soc UK 95:487-494, 1975.

97. Zimmerman LE, McLean IW: Do growth and onset of symptoms of uveal melanomas indicate subclinical metastasis? Ophthalmology 91:685-691, 1984.

CHAPTER 2

DIAGNOSTIC STUDIES

Several studies can assist in diagnosing a malignant melanoma. However, in most cases, skilled ultrasonography and well-resolved fluorescein angiography provide sufficient information and are the studies most commonly used.

ULTRASONOGRAPHY

Ultrasonography is an essential tool in the diagnosis and management of malignant melanoma.[24,31,42,69,101,130,131] Diagnosis of a tumor with ultrasonography is most accurate when the mass has a height of a least 2.0 mm.[18,19,45,47,63,102] Ultrasonography is also invaluable for management of malignant melanoma because accurate and objective assessment of the apical height of a melanoma is possible.[24,42,63,69,101,102] Additionally, ultrasonography can determine if extraocular tumor extension is present.[15,13,45,47,63,102] Ultrasonography is also essential for complete evaluation of an eye with opaque media.[22,31,42,53,63,69,101] When opaque media preclude ophthalmoscopic examination of the retina, the possibility of an unrecognized tumor should be evaluated with ultrasonography.[27,109,135]

Ultrasound examination[29–31,42,63,69,101,130] is performed optimally with both standardized contact A-scan and B-scan instruments. A-scan provides one-dimensional assessment of tissue characteristics and apical height, while B-scan produces a two-dimensional image to assess gross elevation and basal diameters and shape. For many people, B-scan images are easier to interpret because of this cross-sectional view. Yet, B-scan examination alone is often not sufficient to make a secure diagnosis, and standardized A-scan evaluation is essential.

Ultrasound echoes occur when the ultrasound beam strikes an acoustic interface.[30,42,63,101,116] The normal vitreous is homogeneous and mostly echo-free; the tumor surface (retinal-tumor interface) is dense and thus produces a distinct echo. Malignant melanomas are highly cellular and their histologic structure is mostly homogeneous. Therefore, they contain few internal acoustic interfaces to produce reflections or echoes. This makes melanomas less reflective than other lesions, such as choroidal hemangiomas, which are very vascular and therefore contain many acoustic interfaces.[69,102] The solid nature of choroidal melanomas attenuates the incident ultrasound beam, weakening the signal as it reaches the deeper layers of the melanoma.[29,31,69,101,120] Moreover, the convex tumor surface can scatter some incident sound waves further weakening the sound beam.[69,102] These echographic characteristics can explain the B-scan and A-scan findings most frequently associated with malignant melanoma.

B-scan ultrasound can best determine the shape of a tumor; a collar-button pattern (**Fig. 2.1**) is classic for a malignant

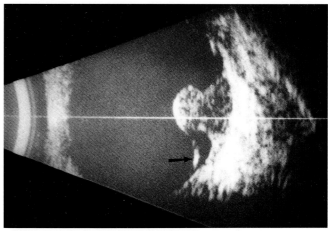

Figure 2.1 B-Scan Ultrasound Of Collar-Button Shaped Malignant Melanoma
This 59 year-old female has an 8.4 mm thick superotemporal malignant melanoma. The B-scan ultrasound demonstrates a collar-button shaped choroidal mass typical of a malignant choroidal melanoma. Note the associated retinal detachment (arrow).

melanoma, but a melanoma may be dome-like (**Fig. 2.2**) or placoid in shape.[31,42,63,69,85] Other characteristic B-scan features associated with malignant melanoma include acoustic hollowing, choroidal excavation and, sometimes, orbital shadowing.[29–31,36,42,85,116,140] Attenuation of the ultrasound beam may produce a more echo-free area (dark appearance on the ultrasound display) in the central, posterior portion of the tumor, called acoustic hollowing (**Fig. 2.2**).[30,31,36,63,69] The dense cellularity and highly homogeneous nature of many malignant melanomas produces acoustic hollowing. Similarly, a somewhat echo-free area in the choroid replaced by the melanoma may create an appearance of a depression called choroidal excavation (**Fig. 2.3**).[30,31,42,69] Occasionally, choroidal hemangioma and metastatic carcinoma show choroidal excavation.[53,102] Variable delineations of acoustic hollowing and choroidal excavation occur when different ultrasound examination frequencies are used. The use of several examination frequencies is believed by some to improve differentiation of a malignant melanoma from other lesions.

Sound attenuation in the orbital tissue behind a choroidal melanoma may produce orbital shadowing.[31,42,69] Extraocular tumor extension may be present if B-scan ultrasound shows irregularities in the contour of the globe wall behind the tumor, or if nodular areas of homogeneity within the adjacent orbital fat are present, or if increasing orbital shadowing is noted with serial examinations (**Fig. 2.4**).[13,15,45,47,119] A careful evaluation for possible extraocular tumor extension should always be done.

A-scan echography can determine if a mass is solid. In the case of a nonsolid mass, small movements of the eye will produce continued movement (aftermovement) of the tracing when the eye stops moving, whereas solid lesions have little if any aftermovement.[42,63,69,101] Vascularity of the tumor may be demonstrated by the observation of fine, spontaneous, fast and

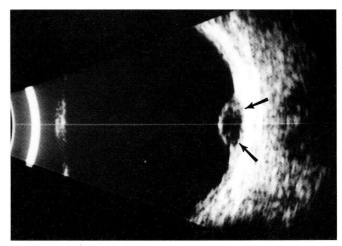

Figure 2.3 B-Scan Ultrasound And Choroidal Excavation In Malignant Melanoma
This 57 year-old has a 3.2 mm dome-shaped choroidal melanoma that shows choroidal excavation (arrows).

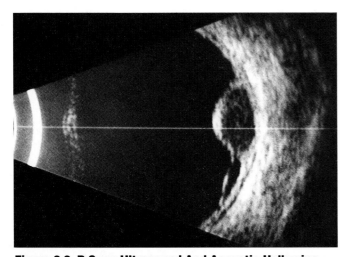

Figure 2.2 B-Scan Ultrasound And Acoustic Hollowing In Malignant Melanoma
This 31 year-old male has a 5.7 mm dome-shaped malignant melanoma just temporal to his left fovea. This B-scan ultrasound demonstrates a dome-shaped lesion. Note that the tumor appears dark because of attenuation of the sound waves within the tumor. This appearance is called acoustic hollowing.

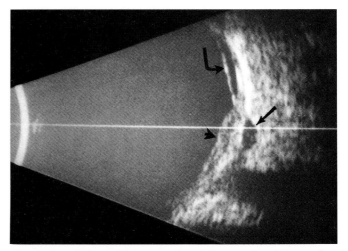

Figure 2.4 B-Scan Ultrasound And Extrascleral Extension
Thirteen years earlier, this 79 year-old female was noted to have a 5 × 5 mm slightly thickened choroidal nevus. She was followed and growth was noted 13 years later. The B-scan ultrasound shows a choroidal mass elevated 2.4 mm (arrowhead). A shallow retinal detachment was also found (curved arrow). Extrascleral extension was documented (straight arrow). The optic nerve shadow can be seen just below. The area of extrascleral extension was further confirmed by orbital CT scan (see Figure 2.12) and at the time of enucleation (see Figure 8.1).

constantly moving vertical oscillations of individual tumor spikes.[30,42,53,63,69,101] These are seen on the video display screen of the instrument and are observed in 70% to 80% of malignant melanomas.[53]

On standardized A-scan, the retina produces a prominent reflection or spike that is maximally high and steeply rising when the probe is oriented perpendicular to the retinal surface.[42,63,69] The height of the internal tumor spikes are lower in the central portion of the tumor than the initial surface spike of the tumor. As one looks from left to right on the A-scan tracing, the height of the ultrasound echoes from the tumor decreases. A low-to-medium reflectivity is characteristic of melanomas (**Fig. 2.5, 2.6**) and varies between approximately 10% to 60% of the initial tumor spike height.[42,63,101,102,140] Reflectivity, however, may be higher and more variable in large tumors.[62,63] Angle kappa is the angle of a line drawn through the peaks of the tumor spikes to the horizontal (baseline) (**Fig. 2.7**).[101] Although not always present, a progressive decrease in height of the echoes from the deeper portion of the mass is characteristic of a melanoma.[94,101,120] Additionally, the height of the internal spikes (reflections) from a melanoma on standardized A-scan tend to be similar. This similarity of the height of the internal tumor spikes is due to the mostly homogeneous nature of melanomas. Tumor necrosis or hemorrhage can increase echo reflectivity and may cause variability of the height of the internal tumor echoes.[22,52,85] The increase in reflectivity alters the angle kappa.

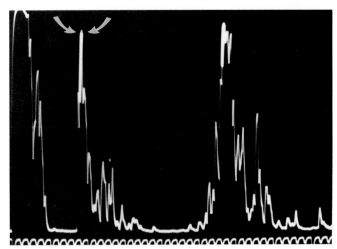

Figure 2.6 A-Scan Ultrasound Of Large Malignant Melanoma

This 60 year-old male noted reduced vision in his left eye for 2 months. He was found to have a large choroidal pigmented mass. This melanoma is large and therefore the ultrasound echo from the retinal-tumor interface is much further to the left than in Figure 2.5 (arrows). The height of the echoes from within the tumor are well below half the height of the retinal-tumor interface echo. This reflectivity of this malignant melanoma is very low. The maximal thickness was 14.8 mm.

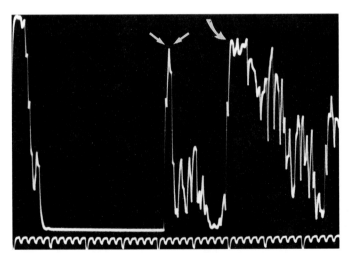

Figure 2.5 A-Scan Ultrasound Of Malignant Melanoma

This 62 year-old male noted blurred vision in his right eye. A posterior choroidal pigmented mass was noted. Note the tall ultrasound echo in the middle of the photo (straight arrows). This is the echo from the retinal-tumor interface. Looking to the right, the next tall echo is from the sclera (curved arrow). The echoes between these two tall peaks represent the echoes from the melanoma. The height of these echoes are all less than half of the tall echoes and mostly similar in height. This is low-to-medium and regular reflectivity that is characteristic of malignant melanoma. The distance between the two tall peaks is used to determine the thickness of the tumor and in this case measured 7.0 mm.

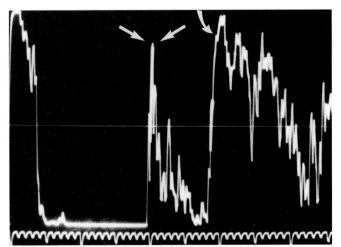

Figure 2.7 A-Scan Ultrasound Of Malignant Melanoma With Positive Angle Kappa

This 31 year-old male with blurred vision in his left eye was found to have a pigmented choroidal mass under his macula. The tall ultrasound echo in the center of the photo is from the retinal-tumor interface (straight arrows). The next very tall ultrasound echo is from the sclera (curved arrow). The ultrasound echoes between these two peaks are from the tumor. Note that the height of these echoes are less than half the height of the retinal-tumor interface echo, and also appear to decrease in height as you look from left to right. This is decreasing reflectivity that is called a positive angle kappa. The maximal thickness of this tumor measured 7.4 mm.

A-scan echography is the most accurate method to measure the height of a tumor.[63] Measurement with A-scan echography is accurate and correlates closely with histopathologic measurements. Still, the size of a tumor measured by ultrasound may differ from the size determined from a histopathologic section due to tumor shrinkage during fixation, tumor sectioning not including the apex, and ultrasound measurement of an area other than the apex.[2,24,96]

A technique has been developed for computerized analysis of digitized ultrasonic information that, when correlated with known standards, can yield histologic cell type information.[32] Specifically, malignant melanoma can be differentiated into spindle B or mixed-epithelioid histologic cell type categories. This procedure has been termed an acoustic biopsy. More recently, a correlation has been shown between acoustic parameters derived with this technique and prognosis.[33] This approach may have the potential to provide prognostic information for those patients who will be treated conservatively such as with radiation therapy.

Finally, high-frequency transducers can enhance resolution of anatomic structures and permit excellent imaging of ocular structures. However, high-frequency transducers penetrate ocular tissues poorly, and therefore, only anterior ocular structures are amenable to this approach.

FLUORESCEIN ANGIOGRAPHY

Fluorescein angiography, though not diagnostic, is useful to exclude disorders such as hemorrhage under the retinal pigment epithelium or retina. Additionally, angiography may provide useful information in the evaluation of smaller lesions since some angiographic findings occur more commonly in melanocytic lesions that subsequently grow.[56,57,100,133]

Fluorescein angiographic findings associated with malignant melanoma include early mottled or patchy hyperfluorescence,[41,46,54,67,75,100,110,149,152] discrete pinpoint leakage,[41,49,55,56,58,67,141,147,152] and visible vessels within the tumor that are sometimes called a double circulation (**Fig. 2.8**).[3,25] But, similar findings may be seen in various benign and malignant lesions.[10] Also, the fluorescein angiographic features may vary, depending on tumor size and associated histologic features.[3,41,49,54,55,92]

The most frequently described fluorescein angiographic feature is early hyperfluorescence. This early hyperfluorescence can be mottled or patchy and often occurs because of a combination of retinal pigment epithelial alterations[41,92,134,149] and vessels within the melanoma (**Fig. 2.8B**).[3,25] The fluorescence increases in intensity (**Fig. 2.8C**) and may subsequently coalesce.[46,75,100,122,141] This appearance may be altered by associated findings, such as hypofluorescent areas caused by blockage of fluorescence by heavy tumor pigmentation (**Fig. 2.9**),[90,110,141] subretinal hemorrhage or fluid,[90,110,122,141] retinal pigment epithelial proliferation,

and lipofuscin pigment.[49,92,138] Additionally, some tumors may remain somewhat hypofluorescent because of less superficial tumor vascularity.[92,141] Drusen may contribute to areas of early hyperfluorescence,[56,92] but this fluorescence often decreases in intensity in the later phases of the angiogram. Areas of balloon cell degeneration within a melanoma may fluoresce to a similar degree as other areas of the melanoma or may appear hyperfluorescent and stain late.[8,77,117,121]

Discrete pinpoint areas of leakage in the late arteriovenous phase become visible sometimes. These are most common with less elevated lesions[58,67] and at the periphery of the tumor just within a surrounding border of hypofluorescence.[41,67,98,147,152] They may increase in number and fluorescence in the later phases of the study.[41,49,55,56,58,67,141,147,152] Although choroidal nevi may have pinpoint leaks, the number of leakage points tend to be fewer than seen with malignant melanoma. Multiple pinpoint areas of leakage (**Fig. 2.10**) are most consistent with a diagnosis of malignant melanoma, and suggest a greater likelihood that a small lesion, if observed and not treated, will grow.[56,57] These punctate areas of hyperfluorescence are most likely due to alterations in the retinal pigment epithelium (RPE) or sub-RPE exudation.[55,92] They may change in position over time.

More elevated melanomas show different features than smaller melanomas. Filling of deep vessels within the tumor (**Fig. 2.8B**) simultaneously with the retinal arterioles can produce an appearance of a double circulation.[3,25] This is more visible in less pigmented tumors and is usually most apparent in the collar-button portion of a tumor that has broken through Bruch's membrane.[3,49,55,67,149] Fluorescein dye leaks easily from these blood vessels (**Fig. 2.8C**), which may give them a feathery appearance.[67] Late diffuse hyperfluorescence is typical in these cases.[46,67]

Retinal vascular abnormalities may be associated with malignant melanoma. Common findings include dilated capillaries, capillary nonperfusion, and microaneurysms.[3,16] Fluorescein angiographic evidence of obliteration or obscuration of the retinal arterioles and venules is a good predictor of retinal invasion.[3] A nonfluorescent area where the tumor has invaded and replaced retinal tissue, and surrounding hyperfluorescence due to leakage into the subretinal space and vitreous, may be noted.[49,55,58,110,128] Additionally, the observation of a tumor-retinal vascular anastomosis is predictive of retinal invasion. Rarely, a dilated, retinal vein draining a melanoma may develop a tortuous or beaded pattern.[72]

TRANSILLUMINATION AND RETROILLUMINATION

Some consider transillumination or retroillumination[116,133] a valuable diagnostic test[113] but it has distinct limitations. Mostly, it is of marginal benefit.[71,116] Since both benign and malignant lesions

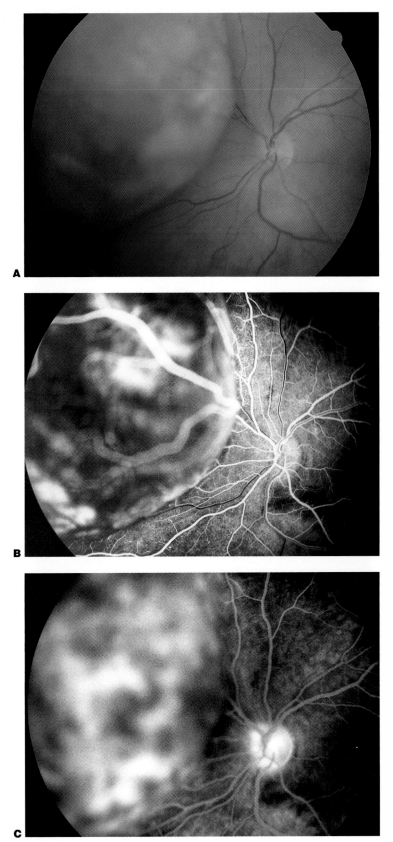

Figure 2.8 A–C Malignant Melanoma and Double Circulation

This 30 year-old female noted cloudy vision for 1 week. The visual acuity in the left eye was 20/20. Note the lightly pigmented medium-sized choroidal mass nasal to the optic nerve (Figure 2.8A). The fluorescein angiogram (Fig 2.8B) showed early hyperfluorescence from within the tumor caused by tumor vessels. There was late leakage (Figure 2.8C) from these tumor vessels in the late angiogram.

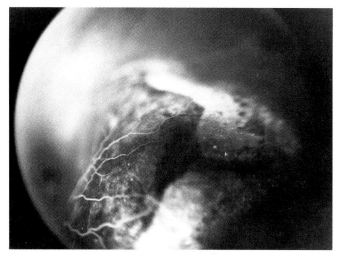

Figure 2.9 Malignant Melanoma With Irregular Fluorescence

This large melanoma has an apical height of 8.4 mm. Note the hypofluorescent areas over portions of this tumor caused by heavy tumor pigmentation compared with the hyperfluorescent areas caused by degeneration of the retinal pigment epithelium.

can produce good or poor transillumination, this test can be misleading. For instance, lesions without pigment, such as metastatic carcinoma, choroidal hemangioma, choroidal effusion, or amelanotic melanoma, may demonstrate good transmission of light.[116,133,154] Alternatively, hemorrhagic retinal detachments and pigmented malignant melanomas will usually produce little transmission of light. Consideration of these limitations is important whenever transillumination is used. If a ciliary body lesion is cystic, transillumination will show good transmission, and if solid, usually poor transmission.[37,133]

Still, transillumination is helpful to assess the size of a ciliary body or anterior choroidal lesion. This assessment may be particularly important for determining management of a ciliary body lesion.[37,133] Transillumination also can be used to estimate tumor diameters for radiation therapy.

There is relatively good correlation between measurements of the basal diameter of melanomas determined by transillumination with measurements made from the gross pathologic specimen or a histologic slide.[112] Yet, transillumination usually yields a significantly larger estimate than direct measurement of the gross or histopathologic specimen. Transillumination is most

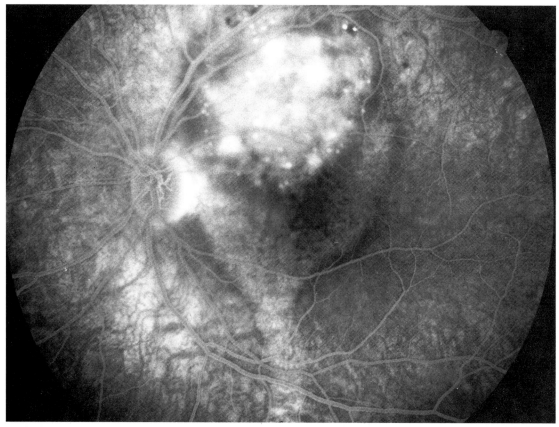

Figure 2.10 Malignant Melanoma With Pinpoint Hyperfluorescence ("hot spots")

This 32 year-old female has a small (7 mm × 7 mm) melanocytic lesion with an apical height of 3.0 mm. Note the multiple pinpoint areas of hyperfluorescence in this late phase angiogram. Also note the track of hyperfluorescence extending inferiorly from the tumor. This is caused by depigmentation of the retinal pigment epithelium from chronic subretinal fluid.

commonly performed by placing the illuminating light source over the cornea and measuring the size of the resulting shadow; therefore, a taller and more anterior tumor will cast a shadow on it's posterior side that will lead to an overestimation of the size. Hemorrhage along the margin of the tumor may cast a shadow and result in an overestimation of size. Tumor shrinkage during fixation and processing can also produce differences in measurements by transillumination and measurements in the pathology laboratory.

RADIOPHOSPHORUS (^{32}P) UPTAKE MEASUREMENT

The original description of radioactive phosphorus (^{32}P) uptake for diagnosing ocular tumors was in the early 1950s.[146] The rationale for this test is that a proliferating tumor will actively absorb ^{32}P (incorporated into DNA), and therefore the tumor can be detected by increased emitted radiation from the area of the tumor compared with noninvolved areas.[26,59] ^{32}P is a beta particle emitter with low energy and shallow tissue penetration (about 3.0mm), characteristics that would tend to be advantageous for a small organ such as the eye.[103,147] As originally used, a conjunctival incision was not made to allow placement of the radiation detection probe directly over posterior tumors. Therefore, except for more anterior tumors, the technique had limited use.[64]

With time the technique was refined: the instrumentation improved, the conjunctiva was incised, and the probe was placed carefully on the sclera underlying tumor.[26,64,123,124,139] This approach produces results with a greater than 95% sensitivity and specificity.[26,59,65,86,95,99,125,129,132,136,147] However, because false-positive and false-negative results do occur, the test is used infrequently today in the United States, though it is still used to some extent in some European countries.[86,98]

The test involves administrating ^{32}P, either intravenously or orally, and measuring the radiation about 48 hours later.[26,43,59,64,86,95,118,123,125,132] It is preferable to compare the amount of emitted radiation over the tumor with the amount of radiation detected from an uninvolved quadrant of the eye rather than with the fellow eye. Calculation of the ^{32}P uptake is according to the formula (CPM equals counts per minute):

$$((CPM_{lesion} - CPM_{control}) / CPM_{control}) \times 100.$$

Usually, a 40% to 65% increase is considered positive,[21,26,59,64,86,99,132,147] whereas others interpret this as indeterminate and look for a greater increase in emmitted radiation.[95,107,125] Results indicate that differentiation of malignant lesions (melanomas or metastatic carcinomas) from benign lesions is accurate.[64,125,132,134,136,147] For instance, it is usually possible to determine the benign nature of a choroidal hemangioma, but there have been some exceptions (false-positive).[34,64,84,93,99,132,147]

However, this test does not differentiate a malignant melanoma from a metastatic carcinoma and false-negative results are frequent with iris, ciliary body, and peripapillary tumors.[26,59,64,118,132,147] False-positive results may occur with such lesions as choroidal nevi, hemorrhagic choroidal detachments, subretinal hemorrhage, staphyloma, scleritis, choroidal osteoma, retinal pigment epithelial hyperplasia, and reactive lymphoid hyperplasia.[86,91,93,129,132,147,153]

Attempts to correlate ^{32}P uptake with certain histopathologic features and mitotic figure counts have shown a relationship in some series,[21,91,114] but not most.[65,107,125,136,147,150] Likewise, it is not definite if there is a correlation with prognosis for survival and ^{32}P uptake.[65,91]

Evaluation of these results reveals that a ^{32}P uptake is an accurate test. Why, then, is it currently used much less frequently? Several factors appear to be involved. Concomitant with the refinement of ^{32}P testing has been the refinement of ultrasonography, which is a very accurate diagnostic method and does not require an invasive procedure.[29] Most lesions can be differentiated clinically with a good accuracy. ^{32}P uptake can not, unfortunately, differentiate a small malignant melanoma from a large atypical choroidal nevus. Differentiation of choroidal melanoma from choroidal hemangioma with ^{32}P uptake is usually accurate, but ultrasonography provides an accurate and easier method. There are theoretical concerns of radiation exposure from the ^{32}P and ophthalmic complications, albeit rare, include subretinal hemorrhage, traumatic episcleritis, and Bruch's membrane rupture.[12,13,19,56,60,118,132,136,147,153]

FINE NEEDLE ASPIRATION BIOPSY

Despite a careful ocular evaluation, including ultrasonography and fluorescein angiography, some intraocular lesions remain a diagnostic challenge. For instance, some patients may have an ocular lesion that suggests metastasis, but they have no known primary tumor despite an extensive systemic evaluation.[4,6,35,38,70] In this difficult situation, obtaining a tissue sample can establish a definite diagnosis.

Many years ago, methods of obtaining intraocular tissue specimens were described but these produced unacceptable local tumor seeding. Fine needle aspiration biopsy (FNAB) has many potential advantages over previously used techniques. FNAB has been used extensively for the diagnosis of many nonocular tumors[50] but experience with this technique for intraocular disorders is limited.[6,19,23,35,38,70] This discussion will be limited to FNAB.

Typically, the eye is entered by passing a small-gauge needle (usually 25 gauge) either through the pars plana or the limbus and directed transvitrealy and transretinally into the lesion (**Fig. 2.11**).[4,19,23,38,70] Alternatively, the eye may be entered by

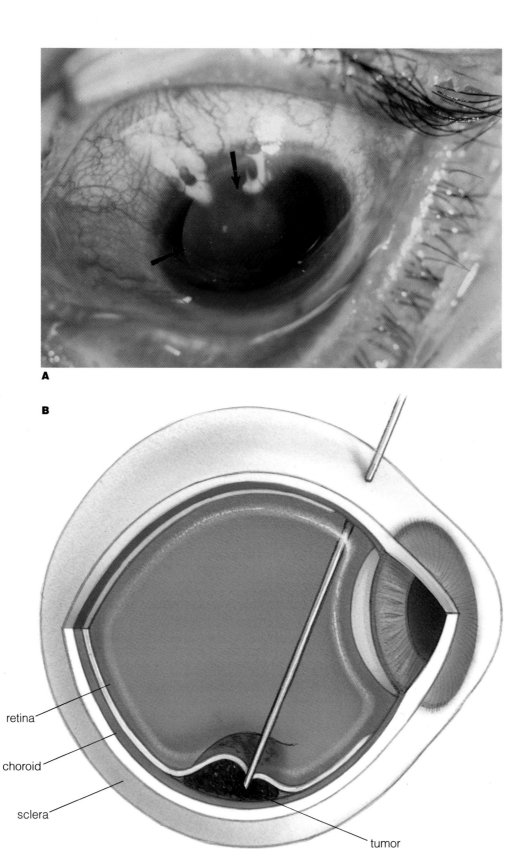

A

B

retina

choroid

sclera

tumor

Figure 2.11A & B Fine-Needle Aspiration Biopsy
A large (16 mm × 16 mm × 10.1 mm) inferior amelanotic mass is present (Figure 2.11A, arrows). A fine-needle aspiration biopsy (FNAB) with a 25 guage needle was done via a transvitreal and transretinal approach. Metastatic breast carcinoma was diagnosed. FNAB can be performed through a pars plana, transvitreal and transretinal approach (Figure 2.11B). This is generally well tolerated with minimal complications.

passing a needle through the sclera underlying the lesion.[4,35] Material is gently aspirated, the needle is withdrawn, and cytologic fixation is performed according to well-described techniques. Essential to the success of this technique is an adequate sample and a cytopathologist experienced with ophthalmic specimens.[6,19]

Some have expressed concern about the potential risk of orbital seeding with this method,[4,70] and there is even some histologic evidence of malignant cells within the needle track.[76] The clinical significance of this finding is not certain, as there is no documentation of orbital tumor recurrence resulting from a FNAB (in contrast with the larger bore needles used previously).[6,19]

Although this technique usually causes intravitreal, retinal, and subretinal hemorrhages, they are usually minor. Long-term visual prognosis is good, and morbidity is minimal. Nevertheless, FNAB of a vascularized, collar-button shaped melanoma may produce substantial subretinal and intraocular hemorrhage.

When reserved for selected cases and performed with the assistance of a skilled cytopathologist, FNAB can yield accurate diagnostic information in over 90% of cases.[6,19,20,35,38,70] Correlation of cytopathologic findings with histopathologic cell classification of malignant melanoma has also been reported in some series[23,35,38] but not in all.[6] Cell culture and DNA cycling studies of cytologic material obtained with FNAB may allow a determination of information, such as mitotic activity, that may influence therapy.[23,78,127] The restricted sample size obtained with FNAB is a limitation; inadequate or nonrepresentative tissue may be aspirated, resulting in false-negative findings.

Vitrectomy surgery offers an alternative approach that may minimize potential ocular complications and possibly obtain a more adequate biopsy sample.[48] The potential for tumor spread secondary to the use of 20-gauge instruments compared with a 25-gauge needle is unknown. Additionally, it is not clear if the potential advantages of this technique are sufficient to replace FNAB.

VISUAL FIELD TESTING

Some investigators have reasoned that differentiation of malignant lesions from benign lesions may be possible with perimetry testing since one could expect more extensive damage to the retinal pigment epithelium and outer retina associated with growing, malignant lesions. Visual field testing, however, is not always reliable for diagnosis.

One potential use of perimetry is to evaluate the extent of field loss associated with a malignant melanoma. In some situations, this may be helpful in counseling a patient, and in other settings, it may assist comparison of different treatment modalities.

RADIOLOGIC STUDIES

With improved resolution of the images generated by computed tomography (CT) and magnetic resonance imaging (MRI), interest has turned toward investigating their diagnostic utility. Although several reports are in the literature, a careful and extensive comparison of the sensitivity and specificity of CT scans and MRI with skilled ultrasonography of various intraocular lesions is lacking.[1,5,17,66,68,87,88,111] One potential advantage of CT and MRI studies is less dependance on the technical skill of the examiner.

Computed Tomography

CT scanning can usually detect lesions as small as 2.0 mm to 3.0 mm in elevation,[1,5,87,111] but less elevated lesions, such as diffuse tumors, may not be imaged.[87] A CT scan shows a choroidal malignant melanoma as a hyperdense mass that is well delineated at its apex by the vitreous cavity.[5,87,111] Contrast enhancement is typical of malignant melanomas and can occur to a variable extent with metastatic lesions.[1,68,111] Choroidal hemangiomas demonstrate a greater degree of contrast enhancement but may not be seen on noncontrast studies.[87] Height measurements from the CT scan appear to be accurate, but basal diameter determinations may be larger than ophthalmoscopic estimates.[5]

Probably the most important role of a CT scan is the evaluation of possible extrascleral tumor extension (**Fig. 2.12**). In some cases, extension of a melanoma outside the sclera may be difficult to detect with ultrasonography. Although the sensitivity

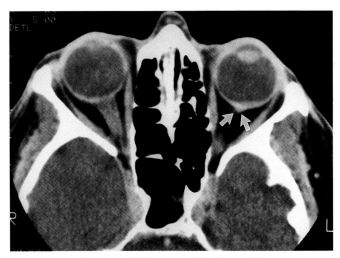

Figure 2.12 Computed Tomographic Scan of Extraocular Extension

This 79 year-old female had a malignant melanoma with confirmed growth. An area of extraocular extension was suspected with standardized echography (Figure 2.4). This was confirmed with an orbital CT scan (arrows).

of detection of extrascleral extension of a malignant melanoma with a CT scan is not known, CT scanning may provide additional supportive evidence.[1,68,87]

Magnetic Resonance Imaging

MRI studies using surface coils have improved the imaging ability of this modality.[7,17,82,151] The paramagnetic properties of melanin provide unique imaging characteristics of ocular melanomas compared with other malignancies.[7,17,61,66,82,143]

MRI is a noninvasive technique for obtaining images of biological tissues in a variety of planes. This technique takes advantage of the high concentration of hydrogen atoms present in water and lipids in all biological tissues. An applied external magnetic field can detect the distribution and concentration of hydrogen nuclei in various tissues. This information can then be translated to provide high resolution images of normal and abnormal tissues.

When a magnetic field is applied, hydrogen, like many atomic nuclei, will spin or resonate like a spinning top.[82] An MRI study uses a constant magnetic field. This external magnetic field causes protons to behave like a gyroscope and precess (rotate) at a characteristic frequency (Larmor frequency) around the magnetic field (**Fig. 2.13**).[82] This phenomenon is similar to a child's spinning top that will spin with its axis aligned parallel with the earth's gravitational field. The direction of the spinning protons

is either parallel to the applied magnetic field (as if the top were spinning right-side up) or antiparallel to the magnetic field (as if the top were spinning upside down). The parallel state is a somewhat more stable orientation. This results in slightly more than one-half of the protons aligning parallel with the magnetic field. If the sum of one proton spinning parallel and one proton spinning antiparallel equal zero, a magnetic field applied parallel to the Z axis of an X, Y, and Z axis coordinate system (Y axis horizontal to this line of print, the Z axis vertical, and the X axis oriented such that it is perpendicular to the plane of the page) will produce a net volume magnetization positive in the Z axis (**Fig. 2.13**). If a constant magnetic field is maintained, then the net positive magnetization vector is also maintained and an equilibrium is achieved.

A radiofrequency pulse can be applied to this system, perpendicular to the steady magnetic field. If a radiofrequency pulse is added to this magnetic field at the same frequency as the protons' precessional frequency, the individual protons will gain in energy. An analogy to a child swinging back and forth on a swing can be made: if synchronous energy is put into the system, such as if someone pushes the child in harmony with the swinging motion, then the child will swing higher. If the pushes are applied at a frequency different from the swinging, the system will not gain energy.

Protons manifest a gain in energy in three ways: increasing precessional angulation, parallel protons becoming antiparallel protons, and protons becoming in phase with each other. If enough energy is applied, the number of parallel and antiparallel protons will equalize, and the Z-magnetization vector will become zero. If the radiofrequency pulses stop, there will be a return to a net positive magnetization in the Z axis and a return to the previous equilibrium state at a rate described by the rate constant T_1 (**Fig. 2.14**). This return of positive magnetization is fastest for protons that are present in an environment of large

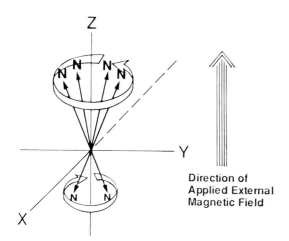

Figure 2.13 Principles Behind Magnetic Resonance Imaging

A three dimensional system is drawn with the Y axis horizontal, the X axis perpendicular to the plane of this page, and the Z axis vertical. The external magnetic field is applied along the Z axis. Each arrow labelled N represents the magnetic moment of individual nuclei. In the presence of a magnetic field, each nucleus will rotate (precess) around this magnetic field (the Z-axis). This rotary movement occurs at a characteristic frequency known as the Larmor frequency. Nuclei above the XY plane are spinning in a parallel manner and those below the plane are spinning in an antiparallel manner. The parallel orientation is somewhat more stable and therefore is more common. This results in more nuclei spinning in a parallel fashion than in an antiparallel fashion and therefore, a net positive magnetization vector.

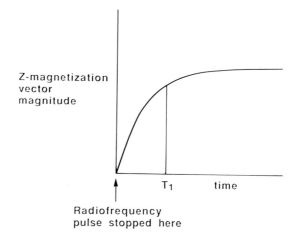

Figure 2.14 The T_1 Rate Coefficient

At time zero (arrow), the radiofrequency pulse is stopped. This results in a return to an equilibrium state with an increase in the Z-magnetization vector. T_1 is the rate constant which describes this increase in the Z-magnetization vector.

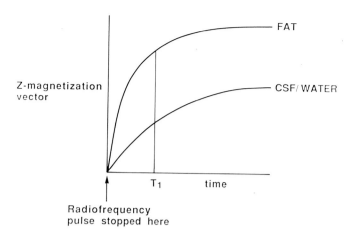

Figure 2.15 Explanation of MRI Characteristics of Different Tissues
Large molecues such as fat have a more rapid T_1 coefficient, whereas, smaller molecues such as water (CSF), have a longer T_1 coefficient. This means that at given time following the cessation of the radiofrequency pulse, more fat molecules have returned to equilibrium than water molecules. Magnetic resonance image generation done as a T_1-weighted image, is a measure of the magnetization vector of a given tissue. If the radiofrequency pulses are applied at a fast rate, then tissues such as fat with a faster T_1, will generate a brighter (whiter) MR image.

molecules such as fat **(Fig. 2.15)**. Small molecules, such as water, have poor energy transfer coefficients and consequently have a long T_1 coefficient. Melanin has unique paramagnetic properties and has a short T_1 coefficient.

Image generation using T_1 as a parameter, that is, a T_1-weighted image, is a measure of the magnetization vector in the Z axis at a given time for a given tissue. If the radiofrequency pulses are applied at a fast rate, tissues with a faster T_1 will yield a somewhat higher signal than will those with a slower T_1. Such tissues as retro-orbital fat will appear bright (white) on T_1-weighted MR images in contrast to more fluid type tissues, such as cerebrospinal fluid, which will appear darker on T_1-weighted images.

A spin-echo technique is used for magnetic resonance imaging of the eye. The spin-echo time is defined as the length of time between the application of the radiofrequency pulse and the moment that the change in the protons is measured (or the echo is listened for) to construct the image.

MRI studies also use T_2-weighted images. For this technique, a radiofrequency pulse is again applied in addition to the magnetic field, but it is oriented from a different direction than that used for a T_1-weighted image. An analogy can again illustrate this parameter. If a group of children begin to swing on a large set of swings, they will be randomly out of phase with each other after a period of time. If each swing is pushed at the *same*

time, each swing will not only gain energy, but in time, the phase of the swinging will become the same. When the radiofrequency pulse stops, the coherence of phase begins to decay. The loss of phase varies among tissues, and the constant, T_2, defines the rate of decay. Similarly, a radiofrequency pulse applied to protons will not only change their spin states, but their precession will become in phase in the X-Y plane. When the radiofrequency pulse stops, the coherence of phase begins to decay.

T_2 is a value describing how homogeneous the proton environments are in the tissue. Homogenous solids, macromolecules and complex tissues, have short T_2 values. Most liquids, such as cerebrospinal fluid, have long T_2 values.

If image generation is performed using T_2 as a parameter, the spin-echo time, or TE, is longer. The time between the applied radiofrequency pulse and the sampling time is longer with a T_2-weighted image than for a T_1-weighted image. Therefore, tissues with longer T_2 values will have high signals and appear white on the image. An MRI study of the brain using T_2 as a parameter, that is, a T_2-weighted study, will result in the CSF appearing white and the lipid-filled brain appearing dark. By adjusting the pulse sequences, one can accentuate and take advantage of differences in hydrogen density, that is, T_1 and T_2 values of different tissues. These can then be translated into differences on gray scale images and produce anatomic resolution and reconstruction.

As with CT scan, MRI has a limited ability to image intraocular lesions less than 3.0 mm high.[40,88] The unique paramagnetic properties of melanin result not only in a short T_1 but also a short T_2. Choroidal melanomas are usually isointense to hyperintense compared with the vitreous or white matter on T_1-weighted images and somewhat hypointense on T_2-weighted images.[11,17,61,88,115,142,143] Others describe less consistent patterns.[66] Little is known about the MRI characteristics of amelanotic melanomas, but some data suggest that an amelanotic melanoma may have T_1 and T_2 features similar to other nonpigmented tumors.[61,115] Gadolinium contrast may provide better visualization of amelanotic melanomas.[11] Inconsistent features of metastatic carcinoma and choroidal hemangioma have been described as well.[66] Metastatic lesions may appear hyperintense on T_1- and T_2-weighted images,[17,88] and choroidal hemangiomas may appear hypointense on T_1 and hyperintense on T_2.[88] Extrascleral extension may be visualized,[40,88,115] and MRI may be more sensitive than CT.

Recent experimental work investigating the use of sodium-23 MRI of malignant melanoma suggests that complimentary diagnostic information may be obtained with proton and sodium-23 MRI studies, and possibly, information about tumor viability.[80] Other experimental investigations of phosphorous-31 nuclear magnetic resonance spectroscopy of malignant melanoma in enucleated eyes have demonstrated that this technique may provide additional diagnostic information and tumor viability data.[81,82]

MISCELLANEOUS STUDIES

Electro-Oculography

The diagnostic accuracy of electro-oculography (EOG) in an eye with a malignant melanoma or choroidal nevi has been studied to a limited extent. Reported studies have compared the EOG (light-peak to dark-trough ratio) of an eye with a malignant melanoma or a choroidal nevus with the EOG of the fellow eye of a patient and with the EOG of an eye in a normal person. The EOG ratio appears to differ significantly in most eyes with malignant melanoma compared with eyes with choroidal nevi.[73,89,144] Also, the EOG ratio of an eye with a melanoma differs from the unaffected fellow eye. The range of EOG test results in fellow eyes can overlap the EOG test results of eyes with malignant melanoma.[89,144] Therefore, there is not an EOG test result that is diagnostic of malignant melanoma.[73,89] The sensitivity of EOG testing is not known. Eyes with a choroidal nevus have a similar EOG as the unaffected fellow eye of the patient.[89]

The reason for the reduction of the EOG ratio in eyes with a malignant melanoma is not clear; the reduction is not explained by the extent of associated retinal detachment.[89,144] These EOG findings seem independent of tumor size.[73,89,144]

Photographic Techniques

Photography with Ektachrome Infrared Aero film can accentuate the brown-black color of melanin and alter the red color of blood to a yellowish hue.[106,145] Although this photographic method is technically more demanding than standard fundus photography, the sharper delineation of tumor margins may be beneficial in following the growth of lesions suspected of being malignant melanomas.[106] Detecting small amounts of melanin within a lesion may help differentiate a less pigmented malignant melanoma from a metastatic lesion.[145] Unfortunately, this technique does not help distinguish a large nevus from a small melanoma. Moreover, large clinical studies have not yet evaluated this technique.[133]

Another diagnostic method that has been studied is absorption differences of infrared light by various lesions.[106] Choroidal melanomas, on average, absorb more infrared light than do choroidal nevi, disciform lesions, or metastatic tumors. However, the amount of infrared light absorption by choroidal melanomas and nevi can be similar, but long-term follow-up of those nevi with a higher amount of infrared light absorption was not available to assess their growth potential. Therefore, the accuracy of this technique is not known.

Other photographic techniques include the application of various colored filters to help differentiate certain fundus details.[44,74] Red light accentuates melanin and decreases the visibility of hemorrhage. In contrast, red-free light emphasizes the hemorrhage and melanin pigment becomes less visible. Yellow light gives melanin pigment a grayish-brown color, and hemorrhages appear dark red or reddish brown. Although comparison of these techniques with other more commonly used diagnostic techniques is not available, it is doubtful that these techniques provide much additional diagnostic information.

Radioscintigraphy

Various radiolabelled agents have been studied as methods of diagnosing malignant melanoma.[9,51,83,104,105,126] A specially adapted gamma counter is used to detect a radioactively labelled tumor-seeking agent and the tumor. One such agent, thiouracil, results in a false melanin precursor.[51] Drawbacks to these agents include limited sensitivity; in particular, depending on the agent, smaller lesions and amelanotic or less pigmented lesions may not be imaged. Perhaps future technological advances in the detection devices, as well as improved agents, may provide diagnostic information concerning smaller lesions, permit assessment of viability of a malignant melanoma before and after radiation treatment, and assist in the diagnosis of melanoma in an eye with opaque media.

One additional approach uses radiolabelled monoclonal antibodies. The antibody binds more specifically to a target antigen, and the increased radioactive uptake is then detected. Preliminary application of this technique to ophthalmology for diagnosis of malignant melanoma has been reported. [99]Technetium-labelled monoclonal antibody fragments to cutaneous melanoma were used in a series of 10 patients.[10] Four patients had pathologically confirmed malignant melanoma, two had presumed melanomas (one of which grew during observation), two had choroidal hemangiomas, and one had a metastatic lesion. Good specificity and sensitivity were demonstrated. The ability, however, of this diagnostic modality to predict growth potential of small melanocytic lesions is not known.

S-100 Protein

S-100 protein is expressed by most choroidal melanomas and is identified in other ocular structures such as Müller cells.[28] Nevertheless, attempts to detect S-100 protein in the aqueous, vitreous, and subretinal fluid in eyes with malignant melanoma, retinal detachments, as well as normal eyes, demonstrated significant overlap in detected levels. This approach, therefore, has limited usefulness.[28]

SUMMARY

Many tests are available that may assist with confirming a diagnosis. In routine practice of ocular oncology, fluorescein angiography and ultrasonography are used most frequently and in general provide all of the information necessary for a secure diagnosis. Additional imaging studies, such as CT scan, may be informative in cases such as suspected extraocular extension. Finally, fine needle aspiration biopsy can usually provide a tissue diagnosis if there is doubt as to the diagnosis. Other studies may become refined in the future to provide still more diagnostic or tissue viability data.

REFERENCES

1. Alsbirk KE, Halaburt H: Computed tomography of malignant melanomas of the choroid. Acta Ophthalmol 61:1087-1098, 1983.

2. Augsburger JJ, Gamel JW, Bailey RS, et al.: Accuracy of clinical estimates of tumor dimensions. A clinical-pathological correlation study of posterior uveal melanomas. Retina 5:26-29, 1985.

3. Augsburger JJ, Golden MI, Shields JA: Fluorescein angiography of choroidal malignant melanomas with retinal invasion. Retina 4:232-241, 1984.

4. Augsburger JJ, Shields JA: Fine needle aspiration biopsy of solid intraocular tumors: indications, instrumentation and techniques. Ophthalmic Surg 15:34-40, 1984.

5. Augsburger JJ, Peyster RG, Markoe AM, et al.: Computed tomography of posterior uveal melanomas. Arch Ophthalmol 105:1512-1516, 1987.

6. Augsburger JJ, Shields JA, Folberg R, et al.: Fine needle aspiration biopsy in the diagnosis of intraocular cancer. Cytologic-histologic correlations. Ophthalmology 92:39-49, 1985.

7. Bilaniuk LT, Schenck JF, Zimmerman RA, et al.: Ocular and orbital lesions: Surface coil MR imaging. Radiology 156:669-674, 1985.

8. Blodi FC: Pathology of choroidal melanomas. Unusual aspects confusing the clinical diagnosis. Trans Ophthalmol Soc UK 97:362-367, 1977.

9. Boer Iwema R, Oosterhuis JA, Pauwels EKJ: Gamma-isotope scanning with 67-gallium and 99-technetium-citrate in choroidal melanoma. In Lommatzsch PK, Blodi FC (Eds): Intraocular Tumors. New York, Springer-Verlag, 1983, pp 258-262.

10. Bomanji J, Hungerford JL, Granowska M, Britton KE: Radioimmunoscintigraphy of ocular melanoma with 99-Tc labelled cutaneous melanoma antibody fragments. Br J Ophthalmol 71:651-658, 1987.

11. Bond JB, Haik BG, Mihara F, Gupta KL: Magnetic resonance imaging of choroidal melanoma with and without gadolinium contrast enhancement. Ophthalmology 98:459-466, 1991.

12. Boniuk M, Hamill B: The ^{32}P test in the diagnosis of ocular melanoma. I. An unnecessary invasive test. Surv Ophthalmol 24:671-675, 1980.

13. Burton TC: Iatrogenic breaks in Bruch's membrane in choroidal melanoma. Tr Amer Acad Ophthalmol Oto 81:841-848, 1976.

14. Byrne SF: Differential diagnosis of disciform lesions using standardized echography. In Hillman JS, Le May MM (Eds): Ophthalmic Ultrasound, Boston, Junk Publishers, 1983, pp 149-161.

15. Canny CLB, Shields JA, Kay ML: Clinically stationary choroidal melanoma with extraocular extension. Arch Ophthalmol 96:436-439, 1978.

16. Cantrill HL, Cameron JD, Ramsay RC, Knobloch WH: Retinal vascular changes in malignant melanoma of the choroid. Am J Ophthalmol 4:411-418, 1984.

17. Chambers RB, Davidorf FH, McAdoo JF, Chakeres DW: Magnetic resonance imaging of uveal melanomas. Arch Ophthalmol 105:917-921, 1987.

18. Char DH: The management of small choroidal melanomas. Surv Ophthalmol 22:377-386, 1978.

19. Char DH: Clinical Ocular Oncology. New York, Churchill Livingstone, 1989, pp 91-149.

20. Char DH, Crawford JB, Gonzales J, Miller T: Iris melanoma with increased intraocular pressure. Differentiation of focal solitary tumors from diffuse or multiple tumors. Arch Ophthalmol 107:548-551, 1989.

21. Char DH, Crawford JB, Irvine AR, Hogan MJ, Howes EL: Correlation between degree of malignancy and the radioactive phosphorus uptake test in ocular melanomas. Am J Ophthalmol 81:71-75, 1976.

22. Char DH, Howes EL, Fries PD, et al.: Uveal melanoma with opaque media: Absence of definitive diagnosis before enucleation. Can J Ophthalmol 23:22-26, 1988.

23. Char DH, Miller TR, Ljung BM, et al.: Fine needle aspiration biopsy in uveal melanoma. Presented at Advances and Controversies in the Management of Ocular and Periocular Malignancies. San Francisco, December, 1988.

24. Char DH, Stone RD, Irvine AR, et al.: Diagnostic modalities in choroidal melanoma. Am J Ophthalmol 89:223-230, 1980.

25. Charamis J, Katsourakis N, Mandras G: The study of the cerebroretinal circulation by intravenous fluorescein injection. Am J Ophthalmol 61:1078-1080, 1966.

26. Chua J: Value of ^{32}P test in diagnosis of intraocular tumors. In Blodi F (Ed): Current Concepts in Ophthalmology. Vol. IV, St. Louis, CV Mosby, 1974, pp 250-263.

27. Chess J, Henkind P, Albert DM, et al.: Uveal melanoma presenting after cataract extraction with intraocular lens implantation. Ophthalmology 92:827-830, 1985.

28. Cochran AJ, Holland GN, Saxton RE, et al.: Detection and quantification of S-100 protein in ocular tissues and fluids from patients with intraocular melanoma. Br J Ophthalmol 72:874-879, 1988.

29. Coleman DJ: Reliability of ocular and orbital diagnosis with B-scan ultrasound. 1. Ocular diagnosis. Am J Ophthalmol 73:501-616, 1972.

30. Coleman DJ: Ultrasonic evaluation of ocular and orbital tumors. In Reese AB (Ed): Tumors of the Eye. New York, Harper & Row, 1976, pp 332-338.

31. Coleman DJ, Abramson DH, Jack RL, Franzen LA: Ultrasonic diagnosis of tumors of the choroid. Arch Ophthalmol 91:344-354, 1974.

32. Coleman DJ, Lizzi FL: Computerized ultrasonic tissue characterization of ocular tumors. Am J Ophthalmol 96:165-175, 1983.

33. Coleman DJ, Silverman RH, Rondeau MJ, et al.: Correlations of acoustic tissue typing of malignant melanoma and histopathologic features as a predictor of death. Am J Ophthalmol 110:380-388, 1990.

34. Cox MS: Discussion of the two preceding papers. Tr Amer Acad Ophthalmol Oto 79:307-309, 1975.

35. Czerniak B, Woyke S, Domagala W, Krzysztolik Z: Fine needle aspiration cytology of intraocular malignant melanoma. Acta Cytologica 27:157-165, 1983.

36. Dadd MJ, Hughes HL, Kossoff G: Ultrasonic characteristics of choroidal melanoma. Bibl Ophthalmol 83:155-162, 1975.

37. Damato BE, Foulds WS: Ciliary body tumours and their management. Tr Ophthalmol Soc UK 105:257-264, 1986.

38. Davey CC, Deery ARS: Through the eye, a needle: Intraocular fine needle aspiration biopsy. Tr Ophthalmol Soc UK 105:78-83, 1986.

39. Davidorf FH: Treatment of malignant melanoma. Letter to the Editor. Arch Ophthalmol 97:975-976, 1979.

40. De Keizer RJW, Vielvoye GJ, de Wolff-Rouendaal D: Nuclear magnetic resonance imaging of intraocular tumors. Am J Ophthalmol 102:438-441, 1986.

41. De Laey JJ: Fluorescein angiographic aspects of choroidal melanomas. Doc Ophthalmol 7:221-236, 1976.

42. Diamond JG, Ossoinig KC: Contact A-scan and B-scan ultrasonography in the diagnosis of intraocular lesions. In Peyman GA, Apple DJ, Sanders DR (Eds): Intraocular Tumors. New York, Appleton/Century/Crofts, 1977, pp 35-49.

43. Dietze U, Jutte A: The significance of the ^{32}P test in malignant melanomas of the eye. In Lommatzsch PK, Blodi FC (Eds): Intraocular Tumors. New York, Springer-Verlag, 1983, pp 247-250.

44. Ducrey NM, Delori FC, Gragoudas ES: Monochromatic ophthalmoscopy and fundus photography. II. The pathological fundus. Arch Ophthalmol 97:288-293, 1979.

45. Duffin RM, Straatsma BR, Foos RY, Kerman BM: Small malignant melanoma of the choroid with extraocular extension. Arch Ophthalmol 99:1827-1830, 1981.

46. Edwards WC, Layden WE, MacDonald R: Fluorescein angiography of malignant melanoma of the choroid. Am J Ophthalmol 68:797-808, 1969.

47. Farah ME, Byrne SF, Hughes JR: Standardized echography in uveal melanomas with scleral or extraocular extension. Arch Ophthalmol 102:1482-1485, 1984.

48. Fastenberg DM, Finger PT, Chess Q, et al.: Vitrectomy retinotomy aspiration biopsy of choroidal tumors. Am J Ophthalmol 110:361-365, 1990.

49. Flindall RJ, Gass JDM: A histopathologic fluorescein angiographic correlative study of malignant melanomas of the choroid. Can J Ophthalmol 6:258-267, 1971.

50. Frable WJ: Fine-needle aspiration biopsy: A review. Hum Pathol 14:9-28, 1983.

51. Franken NAP, van Delft JL, Bleeker JC, et al.: Scintimetric detection of choroidal malignant melanoma with [^{123}I]-5-iodo-2-thiouracil. Ophthalmologica 193:248-254, 1986.

52. Freyler H, Arnfelser H: Relation between histological structure and ultrasonogram in malignant melanoblastoma of the choroid. Bibl Ophthalmol 83:163-171, 1975.

53. Fuller DG, Snyder WB, Hutton WL, Vaiser A: Ultrasonographic features of choroidal malignant melanomas. Arch Ophthalmol 97:1465-1472, 1979.

54. Gass JDM: Differential Diagnosis of Intraocular Tumors. A Stereoscopic Presentation. St. Louis, CV Mosby, 1974.

55. Gass JDM: Fluorescein angiography. An aid in the differential diagnosis of intraocular tumors. Int Ophthalmol Clin 12:85-120, 1972.

56. Gass JDM: Problems in the differential diagnosis of choroidal nevi and malignant melanomas. Am J Ophthalmol 83:299-323, 1977.

57. Gass JDM: Observation of suspected choroidal and ciliary body melanomas for evidence of growth prior to enucleation. Ophthalmology 87:523-528, 1980.

58. Gitter KA, Meyer D, Sarin LK, et al.: Fluorescein and ultrasound in diagnosis of intraocular tumors. Am J Ophthalmol 66:719-730, 1968.

59. Goldberg G, Kara GB, Previte LR: The use of radioactive phosphorus (^{32}P) in the diagnosis of ocular tumors. Am J Ophthalmol 90:817-828, 1980.

60. Goldfarb DA, Streeten BW: Traumatic episcleritis following ^{32}phosphorus testing. Arch Ophthalmol 98:331-334, 1980.

61. Gomori JM, Grossman RI, Shields JA, et al.: Choroidal melanomas: Correlation of NMR spectroscopy and MR imaging. Radiology 158:443-445, 1986.

62. Green RL: Echographic diagnosis of large choroidal melanomas. In Hillman JS, Le May MM (Eds): Ophthalmic Ultrasonography. Boston, Junk Publishers, 1983, pp 15-20.

63. Green RL, Byrne SF: Diagnostic ophthalmic ultrasound. In Ryan S (Ed): Retina. vol. 1, St. Louis, CV Mosby, 1989, pp 191-273.

64. Hagler WS, Jarrett WH, Humphrey WT: The radioactive phosphorus uptake test in diagnosis of uveal melanoma. Arch Ophthalmol 83:548-557, 1970.

65. Hagler WS, Jarrett WH, Killian JH: The use of the ^{32}P test in the management of malignant melanoma of the choroid: A five-year follow-up study. Tr Amer Acad Ophthalmol Oto 83:49-60, 1977.

66. Haik BG, Louis LS, Smith ME, et al.: Magnetic resonance imaging in choroidal tumors. Ann Ophthalmol 19:218-238, 1987.

67. Hayreh SS: Choroidal melanomata. Fluorescence angiographic and histopathological study. Br J Ophthalmol 54:145-160, 1970.

68. Heller M, Gurhoff R, Hagermann J, Jend HH: CT of malignant choroidal melanoma—Morphology and perfusion characteristics. Neuroradiology 23:23-30, 1982.

69. Hodes BL: Ultrasonographic diagnosis of choroidal malignant melanoma. Surv Ophthalmol 22:29-40, 1977.

70. Jakobiec FA, Coleman DJ, Chattock A, Smith M: Ultrasonically guided needle biopsy and cytologic diagnosis of solid intraocular tumors. Tr Am Acad Ophthalmol Oto 86:1662-1681, 1979.

71. Jensen OA: Malignant melanomas of the uvea in Denmark 1943-1952. A clinical, histopathological, and prognostic study. Acta Ophthalmol (Suppl) 75:1-220, 1963.

72. Johnson RN, Irvine AR, Char DH: Inferences from beading of a retinal vein draining a choroidal melanoma. Br J Ophthalmol 70:764-765, 1986.

73. Jones M, Klein R, de Venecia G, Myers FL: Abnormal electro-oculograms from eyes with a malignant melanoma of the choroid. Invest Ophthalmol 20:276-279, 1981.

74. Jutte A, Konigsdorffer E, Schweitzer D: The value of spectroscopy in the diagnosis of intraocular tumors. In Lommatzsch PK, Blodi FC (Eds): Intraocular Tumors. New York, Springer-Verlag, 1983, pp 203-207.

75. Karel I, Teleska M: Fluorescence angiography in intraocular tumors. Ophthalmologica 164:161-181, 1972.

76. Karcioglu ZA, Gordon RA, Karcioglu GL: Tumor seeding in ocular fine needle aspiration biopsy. Ophthalmol 92:1763-1767, 1985.

77. Khalil MK: Balloon cell malignant melanoma of the choroid: Ultrastructural studies. Br J Ophthalmol 67:579-584, 1983.

78. Kindy-Degnan NA, Char DH, Castro JR, et al.: Effect of various doses of radiation for uveal melanoma on regression, visual acuity, complications, and survival. Am J Ophthalmol 107:114-120, 1989.

79. Knobel HH: A clinical report on infrared photography for the differential diagnosis and follow-up of choroidal tumors. In Lommatzsch PK, Blodi FC (Eds): Intraocular Tumors. New York, Springer-Verlag, 1983, pp 199-202.

80. Kolodny NH, Gragoudas ES, D'Amico DJ, et al.: Proton and sodium 23 magnetic resonance imaging of human ocular tissues. A model study. Arch Ophthalmol 105:1532-1536, 1987.

81. Kolodny NH, Gragoudas ES, D'Amico DJ, et al.: Preliminary results on phosphorus-31 nuclear magnetic resonance evaluation of human uveal melanoma in enucleated eyes. Ophthalmology 95:666-673, 1988.

82. Kolodny NH, Gragoudas ES, D'Amico DJ, Albert DM: Magnetic resonance imaging and spectroscopy of intraocular tumors. Surv Ophthalmol 33:502-514, 1989.

83. Lambrecht RM, Packer S, Wolf A, et al.: Detection of ocular melanoma with 4-(3-dimethylaminopropylamino)-7-[^{123}I]-iodoquinoline. J Nucl Med 25:800-804, 1984.

84. Lanning R, Shields JA: Comparison of radioactive phosphorus (^{32}P) uptake test in comparable sized choroidal melanomas and hemangiomas. Am J Ophthalmol 87:769-772, 1979.

85. Lin DTC, Munk PL, Maberley AL, et al.: Ultrasonography of pathologically proved choroidal melanoma with a high-resolution small-parts scanner. Can J Ophthalmol 22:161-164, 1987.

86. Lommatzsch PK, Correns HJ, Rudolph JM, et al.: The reliability of radioactive phosphorous (^{32}P) in the diagnosis of intraocular tumors; Experience with 912 patients. In Lommatzsch PK, Blodi FC (Eds): Intraocular Tumors. New York, Springer-Verlag, 1983, pp 239-246.

87. Mafee MF, Peyman GA, McKusick MA: Malignant uveal melanoma and similar lesions studied by computed tomography. Radiology 156:403-408, 1985.

88. Mafee MF, Peyman GA, Peace JH, et al.: Magnetic resonance imaging in the evaluation and differentiation of uveal melanoma. Ophthalmology 94:341-348, 1987.

89. Markoff JI, Shakin E, Shields JA, Augsburger JJ: The electro-oculogram in eyes with choroidal melanoma. Ophthalmology 88:1122-1125, 1981.

90. McKelvey JAW, Rosen ES, Lucas DR: Photographic methods in the diagnosis of choroidal malignant melanomata. Tr Ophthalmol Soc UK 93:103-106, 1973.

91. McLean IW, Shields JA: Prognostic value of ^{32}P uptake in posterior uveal melanomas. Ophthalmology 87:543-548, 1980.

92. McMahon RT, Tso MOM, McLean IW: Histologic localization of sodium fluorescein in choroidal malignant melanomas. Am J Ophthalmol 83:836-846, 1977.

93. Minckler D, Font RL, Shields JA: Non-melanoma ocular lesions with positive ^{32}P tests. In Jakobiec F (Ed): Ocular and Adnexal Tumors. Birmingham, Aesculapius Publishers, 1978, pp 245-256.

94. Minning CA, Davidorf FH: Ossoinig's angle of ultrasonic absorption and its role in the diagnosis of malignant melanoma. Ann Ophthalmol 14:564-568, 1982.

95. Moseley H, Foulds WS: Observations on the ^{32}P uptake test. Br J Ophthalmol 64:186-190, 1980.

96. Nicholson DH, Frazier-Byrne S, Chieu MT, et al.: Echographic and histologic tumor height measurements in uveal melanoma. Am J Ophthalmol 100:454-457, 1985.

97. Norton EWD, Gutman F: Fluorescein angiography and hemangiomas of the choroid. Arch Ophthalmol 78:121-125, 1967.

98. Oosterhuis JA, De Wolf-Rouendaal D: Differential diagnosis of very small melanomas and naevi of the choroid. In Oosterhuis JA (Ed): Ophthalmic Tumors. Dordrecht, Junk Publishers, 1985, pp 1-8.

99. Oosterhuis JA, Pauwels EKJ, de Wolff-Rouendaal D, et al.: ^{32}Phosphorus uptake test in choroidal melanomas, naevi and haemangiomas. Doc Ophthalmol 50:9-19, 1980.

100. Oosterhuis JA, Van Waveren GW: Fluorescein photography in malignant melanoma. Ophthalmologica 156:101-116, 1968.

101. Ossoinig KC, Bigar R, Kaefring SL: Malignant melanoma of the choroid and ciliary body. A differential diagnosis in clinical echography. Bibl Ophthalmol 83:141-154, 1975.

102. Ossoinig KC, Harrie RP: Diagnosis of intraocular tumors with standardized echography. In Lommatzsch PK, Blodi FC (Eds): Intraocular Tumors. New York, Springer-Verlag, 1983, pp 154-175.

103. Packer S: Radioactive phosphorus for the detection of ocular melanomas. Arch Ophthalmol 90:17-20, 1973.

104. Packer S, Lambrecht RM, Christman DR, et al.: Metal isotopes used as radioactive indicators of ocular melanoma. Am J Ophthalmol 83:80-94, 1977.

105. Packer S, Lambrecht RM, Fairchild RG, et al.: Non-invasive nuclear detection of choroidal melanoma. In Lommatzsch PK, Blodi FC (Eds): Intraocular Tumors. New York, Springer-Verlag, 1983, pp 227-234.

106. Packer S, Schneider K, Hong-Zen L, Feldman M: Digital infrared fundus reflectance. Ophthalmol 87:534-542, 1980.

107. Packer S, Shields JA, Christman DR, et al.: Radioactive phosphorus uptake test. An in vitro analysis of choroidal melanoma and ocular tissues. Invest Ophthalmol 19:386-392, 1980.

108. Pavlin CJ, Harasiewicz K, Sherar MD, Foster FS: Clinical use of ultrasound biomicroscopy. Ophthalmology 98:287-295, 1991.

109. Pe'er J, Savino DF, McLean IW, Zimmerman LE: Posterior uveal melanomas in aphakic and pseudophakic eyes. Am J Ophthalmol 101:458-460, 1986.

110. Pettit TH, Barton A, Foos RY, Christensen RE: Fluorescein angiography of choroidal melanomas. Arch Ophthalmol 83:27-38, 1970.

111. Peyster RG, Augsburger JJ, Shields JA, et al.: Choroidal melanoma: Comparison of CT, fundoscopy, and US. Radiology 156:675-680, 1985.

112. Polivogianis L, Seddon JM, Glynn RJ, et al.: Comparison of trans-illumination and histologic slide measurements of tumor diameter in uveal melanoma. Ophthalmology 95:1576-1582, 1988.

113. Raivio I: Uveal melanoma in Finland. An epidemiological, clinical, histological and prognostic Study. Acta Ophthalmol 133:5-64, 1977.

114. Rao NA, Gamel JW, McMahon RT, McLean IW: Correlation of in vitro ^{32}P counts with histologic features of malignant melanoma of choroid and ciliary body. Invest Ophthalmol 16:98-102, 1977.

115. Raymond WR, Char DH, Norman D, and Protzko EE: Magnetic resonance imaging evaluation of uveal tumors. Am J Ophthalmol 111:633-641, 1991.

116. Reese AB: Pigmented tumors. In Tumors of the Eye. Third Ed. New York, Harper & Row, 1976, pp 173-226.

117. Riley FC: Balloon cell melanoma of the choroid. Arch Ophthalmol 92:131-133, 1974.

118. Robertson DM: Radioactive phosphorus uptake testing of choroidal lesions. A report of two false-negative tests. Br J Ophthalmol 60:835-839, 1976.

119. Rochels R, Nover A: Small choroidal melanoma with diffuse orbital involvement detected and differentiated with standarized echography. Ophthalmologica 192:39-45, 1986.

120. Rochels R, Nover A, Neumann T, Adam F: Echographic examinations on 110 histologically proven intraocular melanomas. In Lommatzsch PK, Blodi F (Eds): Intraocular Tumors. New York, Springer-Verlag, 1983, pp 176-182.

121. Rodrigues MM, Shields JA: Malignant melanoma of the choroid with balloon cells. A clinicopathologic study of three cases. Can J Ophthalmol 11:208-215, 1976.

122. Rubinstein K: Differential diagnosis of malignant melanoma. Tr Ophthalmol Soc UK 87:447-456, 1967.

123. Ruiz RS: The ^{32}P test in the diagnosis of ocular melanoma. II. A reliable and useful clinical guide. Surv Ophthalmol 24:671,676-678, 1980.

124. Ruiz RS: New radioactive detection probe and scaler for phosphorus 32 testing of ocular lesions. Tr Amer Acad Ophthalmol Oto 76:535-536, 1972.

125. Ruiz RS, Howerton EE: ^{32}P testing for posterior segment lesions. Tr Am Acad Ophthalmol Oto 79:287-296, 1975.

126. Safi N, Bockslaff H, Blanquet P, Lerebeller MJ: Non contact detection of intraocular tumors with radionuclides; radiopharmaceuticals, instrumentation and clinical aspects. In Lommatzsch PK, Blodi FC (Eds): Intraocular Tumors. New York, Springer-Verlag, 1983, pp 219-226.

127. Schachat AP, Newsome DA, Miller E, et al.: Tissue culture of human choroidal melanoma cells obtained by fine-needle aspiration biopsy. Albrecht v Graefe's Arch Ophthalmol 224:407-413, 1986.

128. Schatz H, Burton TC, Yannuzzi LA, Rabb M: Interpretation of Fundus Fluorescein Angiography. St. Louis, CV Mosby, 1978.

129. Shammas HF, Burton TC, Weingeist TA: False-positive results with the radioactive phosphorus test. Arch Ophthalmol 95:2190-2192, 1977.

130. Shammas HJ: Atlas of Ophthalmic Ultrasonography and Biometry. St. Louis, CV Mosby Company 1984, pp 57-110.

131. Shields JA: Current approaches to the diagnosis and management of choroidal melanomas. Surv Ophthalmol 21:443-463, 1977.

132. Shields JA: Accuracy and limitations of the ^{32}P test in the diagnosis of ocular tumors: An analysis of 500 cases. Tr Am Acad Ophthalmol Oto 85:950-966, 1978.

133. Shields JA: Diagnosis and Management of Intraocular Tumors. St. Louis, CV Mosby Co, 1983.

134. Shields JA, Annesley WH, Totino JA: Nonfluorescent malignant melanoma of the choroid diagnosed with the radioactive phosphorus uptake test. Am J Ophthalmol 79:634-640, 1975.

135. Shields JA, Augsburger JJ: Cataract surgery and intraocular lenses in patients with unsuspected malignant melanoma of the ciliary body and choroid. Ophthalmology 92:823-826, 1985.

136. Shields JA, Hagler WS, Federman JL, et al.: The significance of the ^{32}P uptake test in the diagnosis of posterior uveal melanomas. Tr Am Acad Ophthalmol Oto 79:297-306, 1975.

137. Shields JA, Joffe L, Guibor P: Choroidal melanoma clinically simulating a retinal angioma. Am J Ophthalmol 85:67-71, 1978.

138. Shields JA, Rodrigues MM, Sarin LK, et al.: Lipofuscin pigment over benign and malignant choroidal tumors. Trans Am Acad Ophthalmol Oto 81:871-881, 1976.

139. Shields JA, Sarin LK, Federman JL, et al.: Surgical approach to the ^{32}P test for posterior uveal melanomas. Ophthal Surg 5:13-19, 1974.

140. Shields JA, Tasman WS: B-Scan ultrasonography of lesions simulating choroidal melanomas. Mod Probl Ophthalmol 18:57-63, 1977.

141. Snyder WB, Allen L, Frazier O: Fluorescence angiography of ocular tumors. Tr Am Acad Ophth Oto 71:820-832, 1967.

142. Sobel DF, Mills C, Char D, et al.: NMR of the normal and pathologic eye and orbit. Am J Neuroradiol 5:345-350, 1984.

143. Sobel DF, Kelly W, Kjos BO, et al.: MR imaging of orbital and ocular disease. Am J Neuroradiol 6:259-264, 1985.

144. Staman JA, Fitzgerald CR, Dawson WW, et al.: The EOG and choroidal malignant melanomas. Doc Ophthalmol 49:201-209, 1980.

145. Suckling RD, Donaldson KA: Detection of melanin in choroidal tumors. Use of ektachrome infrared aero film. Arch Ophthalmol 83:700-703, 1970.

146. Thomas CI, Krohmer JS, Storaasli JP: Detection of intraocular tumors with radioactive phosphorus. Arch Ophthalmol 47:276-286, 1952.

147. Van Dijk RA: The ^{32}P test and other methods in the diagnosis of intraocular tumors. (Thesis). Doc Ophthalmol 16:1-132, 1978.

148. Wallow IHL, Tso MOM: Proliferation of the retinal pigment epithelium over malignant choroidal tumors. A light and electron microscopic study. Am J Ophthalmol 73:914-926, 1972.

149. Wessing A, Foerster M: Fluorescein angiography and the differential diagnosis of intraocular tumors. In Lommatzsch PK, Blodi FC (Eds): Intraocular Tumors. New York, Springer-Verlag, 1983, pp 183-190.

150. Wjollensak J, Heinrich M: In vivo and in vitro measurements of ^{32}P uptake in the ocular tissue in cases of malignant melanoma. Albrecht v Graefes Arch Ophthalmol 217:35-44, 1981.

151. Worthington BS, Wright JE, Curati WL, et al.: The role of magnetic resonance imaging techniques in the evaluation of orbital and ocular disease. Clin Radiol 37:219-226, 1986.

152. Yanko L: An angiographic and histologic study of the vasculature of choroidal malignant melanoma. Acta Ophthalmol 51:12-24, 1973.

153. Zakov ZN, Smith TR, Albert DM: False-positive ^{32}P uptake tests. Arch Ophthalmol 96:2240-2243, 1978.

154. Zimmerman LE: Problems in the diagnosis of malignant melanomas of the choroid and ciliary body. The 1972 Arthur J. Bedell Lecture. Am J Ophthalmol 75:917-929, 1973.

CHAPTER 3

DIFFERENTIAL DIAGNOSIS

The diagnosis of malignant melanoma is made usually with a high degree of certainty based only on ophthalmoscopic appearances. Diagnostic studies, such as ultrasonography and fluorescein angiography, provide additional information and usually secure the diagnosis. An error can occur when an atypical lesion develops that looks and tests similar to a malignant melanoma. A thorough familiarity with commonly confused lesions, both typical and atypical features, is important and increases diagnostic accuracy.

Determination of the basal diameter and apical height of a lesion is helpful for diagnostic and management decisions. For malignant melanoma, lesions are frequently classified as small, medium, or large. A common convention considers a small lesion as less than 10 mm in basal diameter and 2.5 mm in elevation, a medium-sized lesion as 10 mm to 16 mm in basal diameter and 2.5 mm to 10 mm in elevation, and a large lesion as greater than 16 mm in basal diameter and greater than 10 mm in elevation.

LARGE (ATYPICAL) CHOROIDAL NEVUS

A common diagnostic challenge is differentiating between a small choroidal melanoma and a large (or atypical) choroidal nevus (**Fig. 3.1,** page 34, **Table 1.1,** page 2). No clinical features will absolutely differentiate one from the other, but some are suggestive.

Some authors prefer designating a choroidal nevus as a benign melanoma.[19,42,94,110] The term nevoma, instead of atypical choroidal nevus, is applied by some to those lesions in the "gray zone" where clinical differentiation is not possible.[19] For the purposes of this discussion, a nevus or nevoma will be differentiated from a malignant melanoma based on presumed metastatic potential.

Before treatment is done, many clinicians observe these lesions for evidence of growth, because a small choroidal melanocytic lesion has an excellent prognosis for survival (i.e. lack of metastasis). Initial differentiation of an atypical choroidal nevus

from a small choroidal malignant melanoma is therefore more important only to predict future growth and less important in terms of an immediate treatment decision.[18,19,39,41,100,105]

Most choroidal nevi are a slate-grey color, but they may be amelanotic (**Fig. 3.1**) in about 5% of cases.[12,19,108] Size is an important criterion for selecting a melanocytic lesion as suspicious.[48,79,88,100] The vast majority of choroidal nevi are smaller than 7 mm in diameter and 1 mm to 2 mm in elevation.[36,42,52] As a clinical definition, one report defined a suspicious nevus as large as 5 mm in diameter and with an elevation up to a maximum of 2 mm.[48] In one histopathologic study, only 13% of choroidal nevi meassured over 5.5 mm in diameter but ranged up to 11 mm in basal diameter.[84]

Autopsy studies suggest that about 9% of eyes contain a choroidal nevus,[52] though a large clinical series suggested that as many as 30% of eyes contain at least one choroidal nevus.[42] Choroidal nevi usually show no change in size,[62,79,86,121,122] though some may grow slowly and remain benign,[70,79] an observation that is probably more common than previously believed, particularly in younger people.[42]

Three signs that suggest chronicity and therefore a benign lesion are drusen (**Fig. 3.2,** page 35) over its surface, a surrounding margin of hypopigmentation, (**Fig. 3.3,** page 35) and choroidal neovascularization.[19,42,48,84,100] Drusen may be seen ophthalmoscopically overlying up to 50% of choroidal nevi.[48,86] Uncommonly, a pigment epithelial detachment may develop over a nevus (**Fig. 3.4,** page 36). This may give the false impression of a collar-button formation.

Visual field defects are common. In one series, 85% of cases had visual field defects and were more frequently associated with elevation of the nevus.[29,85,86,122] These visual field changes are due to associated choriocapillaris, retinal pigment epithelial and photoreceptor alterations that choroidal nevi may produce, particularly with growth, elevation, encroachment and compression of these structures.[62] But the presence of a visual field defect does not imply future growth of the choroidal nevus, nor malignancy. An absolute scotoma may be produced by a choroidal nevus.[1,19,85,88] Therefore, the determination that a lesion is benign or malignant should not be based on visual field changes.

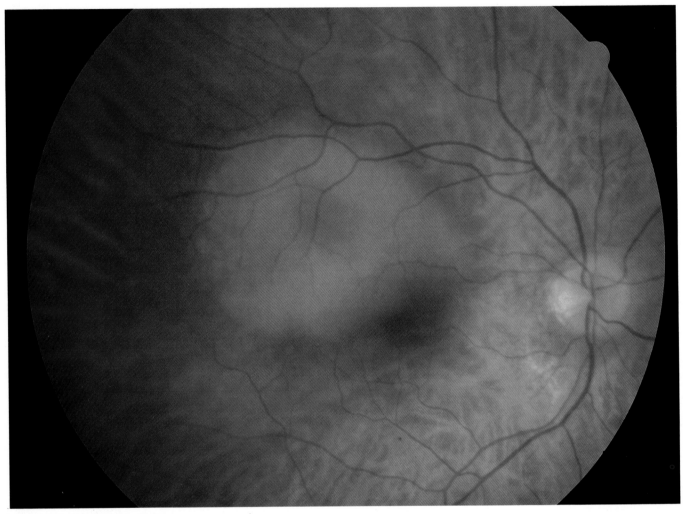

Figure 3.1 Amelanotic Nevus
This 56 year-old female was noted to have an amelanotic nevus 10 years earlier. Visual acuity was 20/20 and no change in the nevus has been observed.

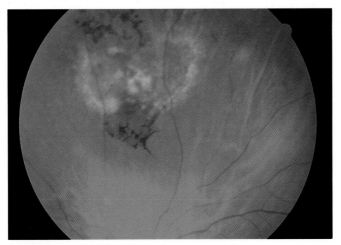

Figure 3.2 Nevus With Drusen and Retinal Pigment Epithelial Alterations
This 70 year-old female was noted to have this pigmented choroidal nevus with multiple overlying drusen and retinal pigment epithelial alterations. Maximal thickness on standardized A-scan echography was 1.4 mm.

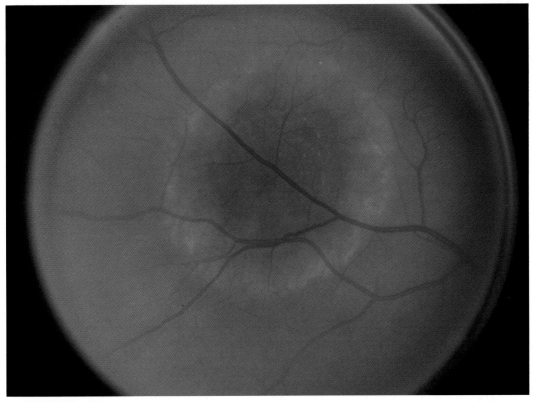

Figure 3.3 Choroidal Nevus With Surrounding Halo
This 46 year-old male was noted to have a choroidal nevus during a routine exam. Visual acuity was 20/40. Note the surrounding area of depigmentation of the retinal pigment epithelium.

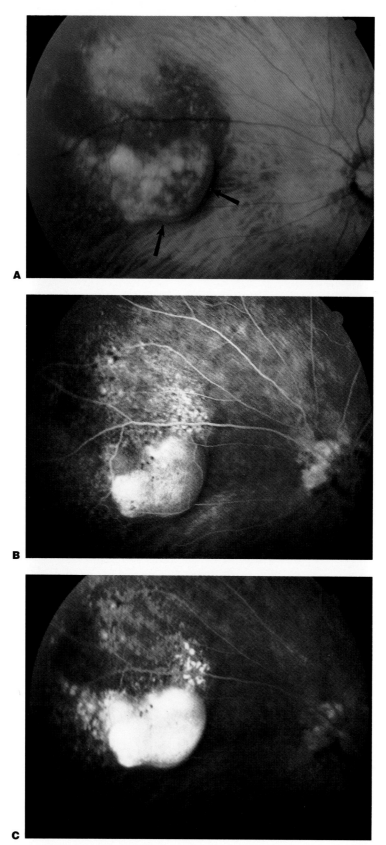

Figure 3.4 A–C Choroidal Nevus With Overlying Pigment Epithelial Detachment

This 63 year-old man was discovered to have an atypical choroidal nevus. An elevation is present along the inferior edge which mimicked a collar-button formation (arrows). The fluorescein angiogram (Figure 3.4B) showed early, diffuse filling of this elevated area typical of a pigment epithelial detachment. Fluorescein pooled (Figure 3.4C) into the subpigment epthelial space but did not leak out of the retinal pigment epithelium.

Features that are suspicious of malignant melanoma include such symptoms as photopsias,[42] some thickness of the lesion or a diameter over 6 mm,[19] multiple areas of orange pigment clumping over the tumor surface,[19,41,108,117] and subretinal fluid (**Fig. 3.5**).[19,42,79] Still, if many drusen are present over the surface of a nevus, subretinal fluid may develop because of decompensation of the retinal pigment epithelium and not tumor growth or tumor activity.[42,79,92] Orange (lipofuscin) pigment clumping has been found only rarely in lesions diagnosed as a choroidal nevus.[117]

Fluorescein angiography of typical choroidal nevi usually shows a somewhat hypofluorescent area caused by pigmentation of the nevus (**Fig. 3.6,** page 38).[54,61,73,91,104] Drusen over the surface may appear hyperfluorescent with little change in the later phases of the study. Pinpoint areas of hyperfluorescence ("hot spots") can occur over the surface of a nevus. A lesion is more likely to show evidence of growth in the future when there are many (more than 5 or 6) "hot spots" present.

HEMORRHAGIC DISCIFORM LESION

Hemorrhage under the retinal pigment epithelium or sensory retina, that is, a hemorrhagic disciform, can appear as an elevated, dark mass (**Figs. 3.7,** page 38 & **3.8,** page 39) and be mistaken for a malignant melanoma (**Table 1.1,** page 2).[26,106,110] A hemorrhagic disciform lesion can occur either posteriorly or peripherally. Rarely, vitreous hemorrhage may be present. Hemorrhage under the pigment epithelium usually appears very dark, whereas hemorrhage under the retina appears more red. Chronic hemorrhage can appear grayish or yellowish due to dehemoglobinization associated with hemorrhage resolution (**Fig. 3.8C**).[43,104] Rarely, the hemorrhage may produce shallow but extensive elevation of the retina. Age-related macular degeneration or other conditions associated with choroidal neovascularization, such as angioid streaks, may produce hemorrhagic disciform scars.[43,104] Examination of the fellow eye may show a similar lesion or earlier stages of the disease process.

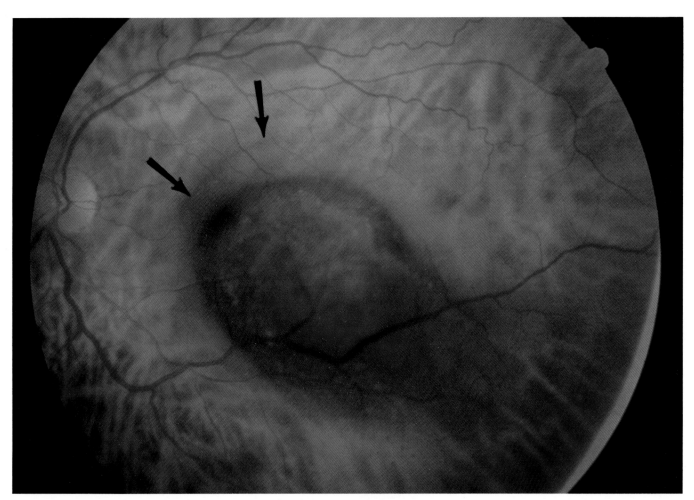

Figure 3.5 Serous Retinal Detachment Associated With Pigmented Lesion
This 46 year-old man was found to have reduced vision in his left eye secondary to a small serous detachment involving his fovea (arrows) that was associated with a pigmented choroidal mass. Note the orange pigment overlying this choroidal mass. This tumor measured 2.7 mm thick.

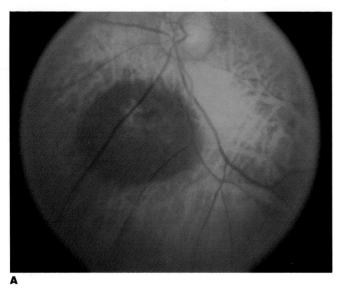

A

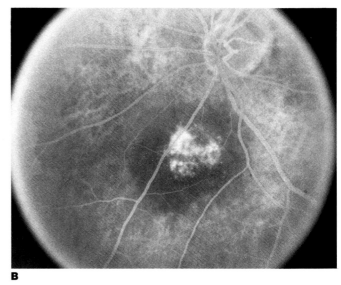

B

Figure 3.6 A & B Choroidal Nevus

This 75 year-old man was found to have a choroidal nevus during a routine evaluation. A late phase fluorescein angiogram shows a hypofluorescent area due to the pigmentation of the choroidal nevus. There is some late staining over the surface of the lesion caused by drusen.

A

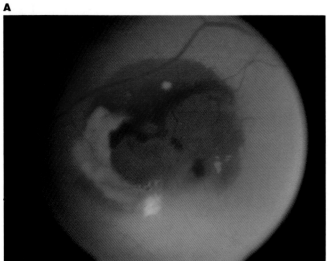

B

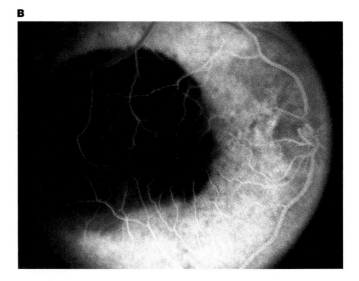

Figure 3.7 A–C Subretinal And Subretinal Pigment Epithelial Hemorrhage

This 75 year-old female developed a sudden reduction in the vision in her right eye to 20/80. A large subretinal and subretinal pigment epithelial hemorrhage was present in the macula. The early fluorescein angiogram (Figure 3.7B) shows substantial blockage caused by the hemorrhage. The hypofluorescence is still marked in the late phase angiogram (Figure 3.7C).

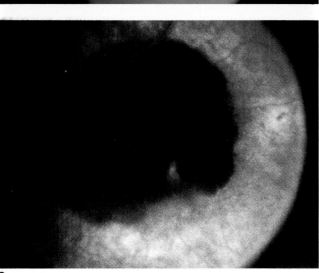

C

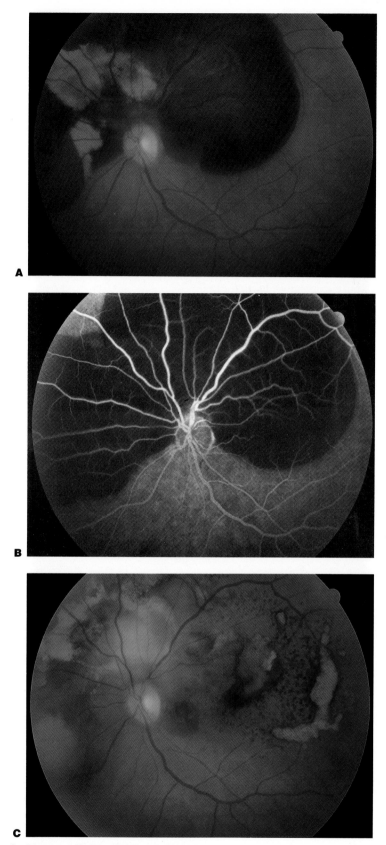

Figure 3.8 A–C Hemorrhagic Pigment Epithelial Detachment

This 72 year-old female presented with sudden loss of vision in her left eye. A large hemorrhagic pigment epithelial detachment is present (Figure 3.8A). Note the extensive hypofluorescence (Figure 3.8B) caused by the subpigment epithelial hemorrhage. Five months later, much of the hemorrhage has resorbed (Figure 3.8C), but some areas of dehemoglobinized (yellow) blood remain. A disciform scar is present just superior to the disc.

Fluorescein angiographic features of a disciform lesion differ from the multiple pinpoint areas of leakage and progressive fluorescence that is frequently seen with malignant melanoma.[30,42,46,54,88,126] A hemorrhagic disciform lesion shows areas of marked hypofluorescence caused by blockage of choroidal fluorescence by subretinal hemorrhage or subpigment epithelial hemorrhage (**Figs. 3.7B, 3.8B**). The choroidal neovascularization may produce visible areas of hyperfluorescence and late leakage may be visible in these cases depending on the extent of hemorrhage.[43,104,108]

Standardized echography can usually differentiate a hemorrhagic disciform lesion from a malignant melanoma.[16,90] When a vitreous hemorrhage is present, ultrasonography is invaluable. A more acute disciform process shows low internal reflectivity. As the lesion becomes more organized, higher internal reflectivity may be noted.[16,90] Since many disciform lesions will contain areas of both fresh and old (organized) hemorrhage, irregular reflectivity may be noted with A-scan echography.[16] In contrast, A-scan echography of malignant melanomas is usually more regular and low-to-medium reflective. Moreover, serial examinations of a hemorrhagic disciform lesion typically proves that the lesion is decreasing in height.[16] Although a ^{32}P test is accurate in differentiating these conditions, it is rarely used.[108]

Despite the differences in ophthalmoscopic, angiographic, and ultrasonographic characteristics between hemorrhagic disciform lesions and malignant melanoma, some may appear very similar. In those cases, observation will usually demonstrate a decrease in size of a disciform lesion.

CHOROIDAL HEMANGIOMA

A choroidal hemangioma (**Fig. 3.9**) can be mistaken for a malignant melanoma.[26,40,55,94,96,101,110,113,116] In a large clinical series, choroidal hemangioma was present in 8% of cases when the referring diagnosis had been malignant melanoma (**Table 1.1,** page 2).[110] An important clue to the correct diagnosis is the characteristic reddish-orange ophthalmoscopic appearance.[40,43,101,130] Two patterns of choroidal hemangioma occur: a circumscribed form approximately 3 mm to 18 mm in diameter and 1 mm to 7 mm in elevation,[4,5,130] and a diffuse form that is characteristic of the Sturge-Weber syndrome (encephalofacial angiomatosis).[5,43,101,130] Most often, a facial angioma (nevus flammeus) occurs with this syndrome. The fundus color of an eye with a diffuse choroidal hemangioma is more reddish than the uninvolved fellow eye and been described as a "tomato-catsup fundus."[43,108]

A choroidal hemangioma may be detected during routine examination or a patient may notice blurred vision caused by subretinal fluid.[4,40,43,108] Ophthalmoscopy may reveal hard exudates, macular pucker, or retinal pigment epithelial and cystic retinal changes produced by chronic leakage of subretinal fluid.[4,5,40,43,101]

Fluorescein angiography is only somewhat helpful in differentiating a choroidal hemangioma from a malignant melanoma.[87,108] Findings include early vascular-type filling of the mass[4,87] with visible large choroidal vessels and a lobular filling pattern (**Fig. 3.9B**).[4,5,43,101,104,108] In the later phases of the fluorescein angiogram, leakage (**Fig. 3.9C**) and evidence of cystic retinal changes may produce a multiloculated staining pattern.[4,5,87,101,143]

Ultrasonography, on the other hand, is very helpful. Standardized A-scan shows characteristic high internal reflectivity (**Fig. 3.9D**), and B-scan shows no significant orbital shadowing.[5,43,101,108,115] Acoustic hollowness and choroidal excavation, characteristic B-scan features of choroidal melanoma (see page 16), are infrequently seen with choroidal hemangioma.[35,108] [32]P testing is accurate in most cases but may produce a false-positive result.[22,51,66,81,89,107,126]

METASTATIC TUMORS

A metastatic tumor in the eye may be mistaken for a malignant melanoma (**Table 1.1,** page 2).[17,26,53,55,94-96,110,113,116,128] Adding to the diagnostic difficulty is the observation that 5% to 10% of patients with a malignant melanoma may have a prior history of nonocular malignancy.[2,28,57,64] Most metastatic lesions to the choroid are carcinomas; breast carcinoma is the most common primary disease in females, whereas lung carcinoma is the most common primary disease in males.[27,34,119,128] Uveal metastasis may be the first indication of cancer in 12% to 46% of cases.[27,34,119] This is particularly true of lung and gastrointestinal primaries, whereas, metastatic breast carcinoma to the choroid is most frequently associated with a prior history of treatment for malignancy.[27,34,119]

A metastatic lesion within the choroid appears as a yellowish placoid choroidal mass (**Fig. 3.10,** page 42). With time, the growing mass and leakage of fluid cause retinal pigment epithelial changes, such as coarse, mottled clumping of pigment, as well as depigmentation (**Fig. 3.11,** page 43).[3,43,128] These pigment alterations can produce a "leopard-spot" appearance. Metastatic cutaneous malignant melanoma may appear as a pigmented choroidal mass, but a preceding or concomitant history of skin melanoma is usually present.[24,32,49,68,119] About 90% of metastatic lesions have subretinal fluid associated with them (**Fig. 3.11**);[34,128] the extent of the subretinal fluid is usually greater than what is typical of a similar-sized melanoma.[119,128]

Metastatic tumors to the choroid occur in the posterior pole region more frequently than other areas;[34,119,128] lesions anterior to the equator account for less than 10% of metastatic lesions.[34,128] Most lesions are less than 4 disc-diameters in size,[34] but some may be diffuse and therefore larger.[43,119] As many as 40% of patients will have bilateral lesions,[3,34,74,119,128] and more than one metastatic lesion per eye occurs in up to 20% of eyes.[34,119,128] Rarely, simultaneous orbital and choroidal metastasis may occur.[15]

A

B

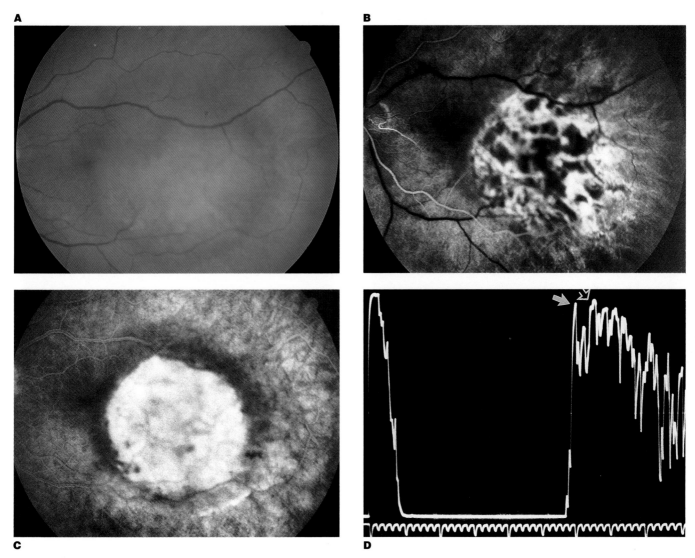

C

D

Figure 3.9 A–D Choroidal Hemangioma

This 66 year-old female noted the recent onset of reduced vision in her left eye. Visual acuity was 20/60. A reddish-orange choroidal mass (Figure 3.9A) is present temporal to the fovea. An overlying serous retinal detachment extends into the fovea. The early arteriovenous phase of the angiogram (Figure 3.9B) shows marked choroidal vascular fluorescence. There is late and diffuse fluorescein leakage (Figure 3.9C) from the lesion. The standardized A-scan ultrasound (Figure 3.9D) shows high internal reflectivity. Note the tall ultrasound echo in the middle of the photo from the retinal-tumor interface (solid arrow). The next echo that is as tall is from the sclera (hollow arrow). The ultrasound echoes between these two peaks are from the tumor and are also very high (high internal reflectivity) that is typical of a choroidal hemangioma.

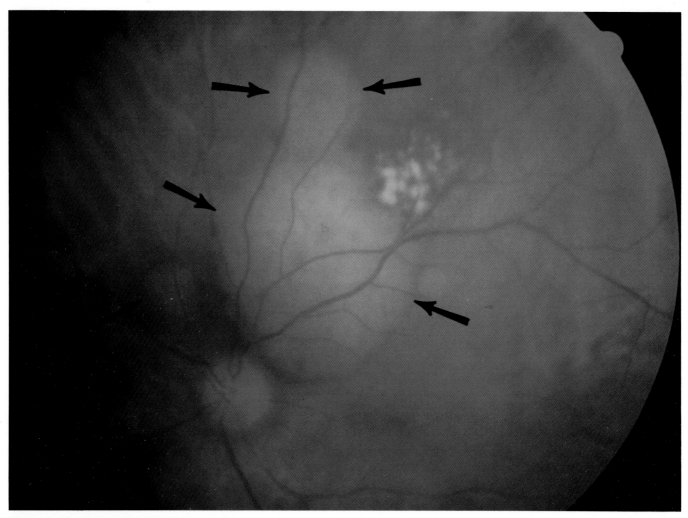

Figure 3.10 Metastatic Breast Carcinoma
This 77 year-old female had a history of breast carcinoma. She noted blurred vision in her left eye. Ophthalmoscopic examination showed an irregular-shaped amelanotic choroidal mass superior to the disc (arrows). Note the incidental finding of a small choroidal nevus with overlying drusen adjacent to the metastatic tumor.

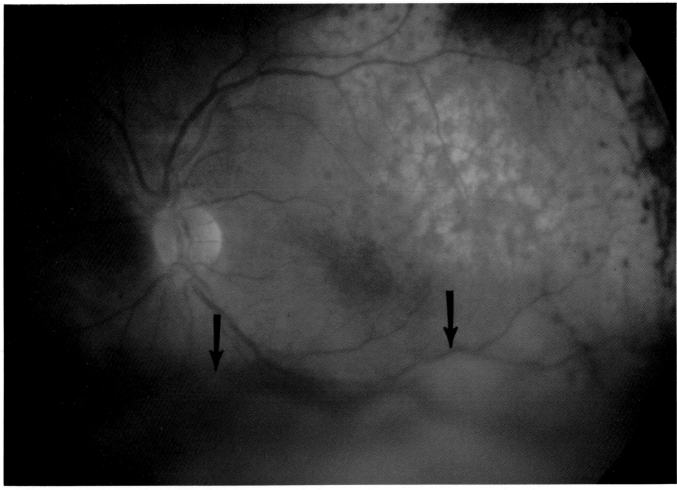

Figure 3.11 Metastatic Breast Carcinoma
This 39 year-old female was on Tamoxifen for metastatic breast carcinoma. Note the choroidal tumor superotemporally with an irregular spotty pigmentation. An inferior retinal detachment (arrows) is present.

Fluorescein angiographic features vary (**Figs. 3.12,** page 44, **3.13,** page 45), depending on the age of the metastatic tumor and extent of growth. New and small lesions confined to the choroid may not be angiographically visible, or they may appear somewhat hypofluorescent.[40] Growth of the lesion frequently produces destructive changes to the retinal pigment epithelium; angiographically, pigment epithelial window defects, blockage of fluorescence by pigment clumping, late staining, and leakage may occur. Angiographic features at this stage may be similar to malignant melanoma.[34,40,43,128]

Standardized A-scan ultrasonography usually shows medium-to-high internal reflectivity (**Fig. 3.14,** page 46) and an irregular internal structure.[82] B-scan examination usually shows a more diffuse or placoid shape rather than the more discoid or ovoid shape associated with malignant melanoma without Bruch's membrane rupture.[21,115] [32]P testing is of no help in the differentiation.[22,47,51,66,81,89,107] Serum carcinoembryonic antigen (CEA) levels are more frequently abnormal in patients with metastatic disease than in patients with a primary uveal melanoma.[20,76,77,78] In one series, 83% of patients with metastatic disease had an abnormal serum CEA compared with 36% of patients with primary uveal melanoma.[78] Additionally, serum values over 10 ng/ml are unusual with melanoma.[20,75,78] Increased serum immune complexes also may be associated with metastatic disease.[20]

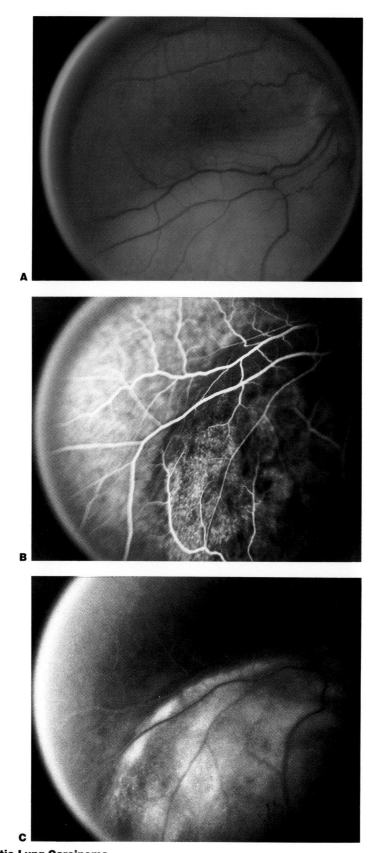

Figure 3.12 A–C Metastatic Lung Carcinoma

This 57 year-old man presented with the recent onset of a "shadow" in his right eye. An amelanotic lesion (Figure 3.12A) was noted inferior to his macula. The early fluorescein angiogram (Figure 3.12B) shows areas of hypofluorescence and hyperfluorescence. There is some late fluorescein (Figure 3.12C) leakage.

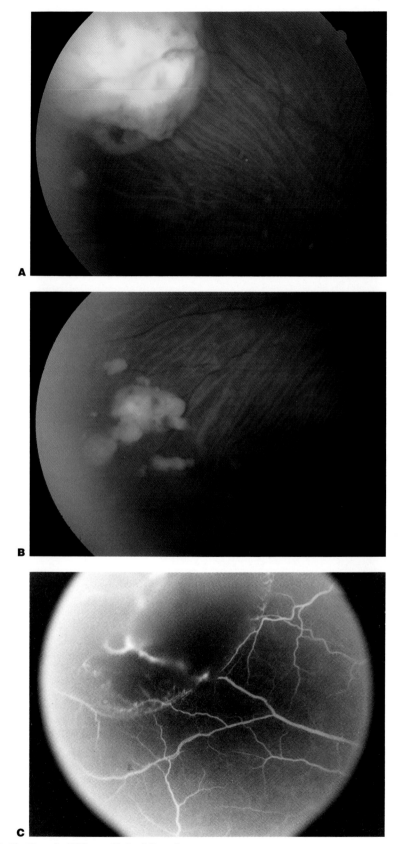

Figure 3.13 A–C Metastatic Poorly Differentiated Carcinoma
This 68 year-old black male noted floaters in his left eye. Visual acuity was 20/40. Several amelanotic choroidal masses were noted with overlying retinal invasion (Figure 3.13A) and vitreous seeding (Figure 3.13B). The fluorescein angiogram (Figure 3.13C) demonstrated hypofluorescence caused by the retinal invasion.

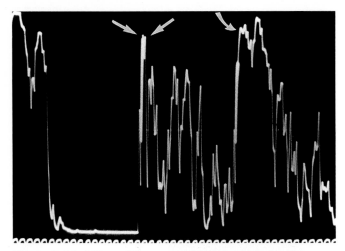

Figure 3.14 A-Scan Ultrasound Of Metastatic Lesion
A 39 year-old female had reduced vision in her left eye secondary to a large amelanotic choroidal mass. Note the tall ultrasound echo from the retinal-tumor interface (straight arrows). The next very tall ultrasound echo is from the sclera (curved arrow). The echoes between these two peaks are from the tumor and are medium to high in height and are irregular. This is typical ultrasound pattern of a metastatic mass.

OTHER MELANOCYTIC LESIONS

Other pigmented lesions that may be confused with a choroidal malignant melanoma include melanocytoma, congenital hypertrophy of the retinal pigment epithelium, reactive retinal pigment epithelial hyperplasia, retinal pigment epithelial adenoma or adenocarcinoma, combined retina-retinal pigment epithelial hamartoma, and benign diffuse uveal melanocytic proliferation.[19,94,108]

Melanocytoma

A melanocytoma most frequently involves the optic nerve (**Fig. 3.15**) but may occasionally occur in the choroid or ciliary body.[59,60,109,111,131] In contrast with choroidal melanoma, melanocytomas are more common in more pigmented fundi as are present in blacks and Asians.[60,131] Patients are generally asymptomatic.[60,131]

An optic nerve melanocytoma has a characteristic jet-black or dark gray appearance with a feathery (fibrillated) distal edge.[59,60] These can extend within the nerve fiber layer of the retina. A melanocytoma may give the impression of optic nerve invasion,[59,108] and subretinal fluid is occasionally observed, as

well.[50,111] Other occasional findings include pigmented cells within the vitreous overlying a melanocytoma,[67] an afferent pupil defect, and visual field loss;[60] none of these findings imply malignancy. A melanocytoma may occasionally be associated with a peripapillary choroidal nevus. When a melanocytoma occurs in the choroid away from the optic nerve, diagnosis may be difficult.[50,109,111] Fluorescein angiography, visual field examination, ultrasonography, and ^{32}P uptake may be compatible for diagnosing a choroidal melanoma.[50,109,111]

Melanocytoma is a benign lesion that requires no treatment.[131] Melanocytomas usually show no ophthalmoscopic changes with time[59,131] but may enlarge in 15% of cases.[59] Therefore, some enlargement of a typical melanocytoma should not be taken as definite evidence of malignant potential. In cases in which the diagnosis is not certain, observation is advisable.[111]

Melanocytoma is simply a variant of a nevus but with distinct histologic features. Melanocytoma has been described as a magnocellular nevus. Histopathologic examination requires bleaching of the specimen to see cellular detail. Melanocytoma cells have benign features; they are large, plump, polyhedral cells with abundant cytoplasm, and have round or oval nuclei and inconspicuous nucleoli.

One unusual lesion has been observed that was initially considered a typical optic nerve melanocytoma but subsequently showed extensive enlargement.[114] Enucleation proved histologic evidence of a malignant melanoma. If malignant transformation of melanocytoma occurs, it is exceedingly rare.

Congenital Hypertrophy of the Retinal Pigment Epithelium

Congenital hypertrophy of the retinal pigment epithelium (CHRPE) is a flat, well-delineated, pigmented lesion with a diameter of 2 mm to 6 mm in most cases.[13,14,65] A surrounding hypopigmented halo is frequently present, as well as lacunae of depigmentation or hypopigmentation within the substance of the lesion (**Fig. 3.16,** page 48). Absolute scotomas may be associated with these lesions and correspond to histologic absence of photoreceptors.[13,14] Transillumination of the globe reveals a well demarcated shadow.[108] Fluorescein angiography does not contribute substantially to the diagnosis since the ophthalmoscopic appearance is generally very characteristic (**Fig. 3.16 B,C**).

This condition may be multifocal and is called congenital grouped pigmentation of the retina, or bear tracks.[43,65] Histologic examination shows increased pigment within the affected cells.[14] CHRPE occurs with Gardner's syndrome (familial polyposis of the small and large intestine).[8,69]

A nonpigmented and newly recognized variant of CHRPE appears whitish (**Fig. 3.17,** page 49); it may occur as a solitary albinotic lesion or as multiple foci and has been termed polar bear tracks.[43]

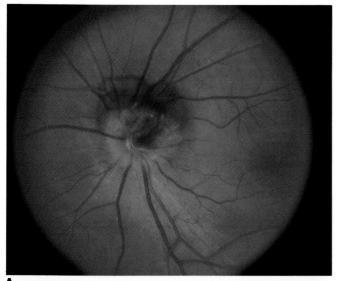

A

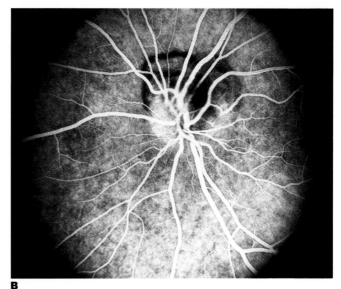

B

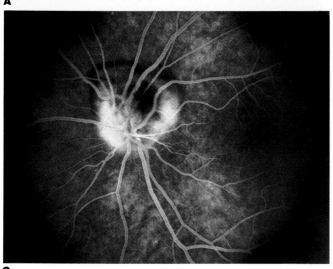

C

Figure 3.15 A–C Optic Nerve Melanocytoma

A 32 year-old female was found to have an optic nerve lesion during a routine examination. The visual acuity was 20/20. Note the pigmented choroidal and optic nerve lesion (Figure 3.15A). The fluorescein angiogram showed hypofluorescence early (Figure 3.15B), with some late fluorescein staining (Figure 3.15C).

through the retina, and onto the surface of the retina. Extrascleral extension of RPE hyperplasia can occur following cryotherapy.[9] This can be mistaken for a malignant melanoma with extrascleral extension. Contraction or shrinkage of fibrous-like tissue within the lesion can cause radiating retinal folds. Fibrous metaplasia of retinal pigment epithelium may produce grayish-white areas over the surface of the lesion.[108] Fluorescein angiography is not especially helpful with the diagnosis. Although ultrasonography can be used to document the extent of the lesion, RPE hyperplasia does not have distinctive echographic findings that are diagnostic.[108]

Retinal Pigment Epithelial Hyperplasia

Reactive hyperplasia of the retinal pigment epithelium (RPE hyperplasia) may occur as a pigmented mass anywhere in the fundus.[65,94,95,110,120,127] In most cases, it is a sequelae of inflammation or trauma, though such a history is not always obtained.[31,40,118,120] Although unusual, somewhat rapid growth may occur.[112] Ophthalmoscopically, RPE hyperplasia is an intensely black lesion with ragged margins (compared with the well-delineated margins of congenital hypertrophy of the retinal pigment epithelium).[19,40,95,108] RPE hyperplasia may look mossy, mottled, or filigreed.[127] Areas of contiguous or distant chorioretinal inflammatory scarring may be observed.[56] RPE hyperplasia may grow and develop a collar-button shape. Proliferation of retinal pigment epithelium may result in growth of RPE into the retina,

Pigment Epithelial Adenoma and Adenocarcinoma

Other tumors of the pigment epithelium, such as adenomas and adenocarcinomas, are very rare and may be impossible to differentiate clinically from a choroidal melanoma.[37,80,106] They can occur peripherally or posteriorly and appear very black.[108,125] An RPE adenocarcinoma, the malignant form of this tumor, is distinguished histologically from the benign variety, adenoma, by local tissue invasiveness, anaplastic cellular features, and the presence of mitotic figures.[37,80] However, some simply designate any tumor of the retinal pigment epithelium as neoplastic.[31,125] Metastatic disease is unusual and has been reported only rarely in surveys of retinal pigment epithelial tumors, and none of these metastases were confirmed pathologically.[37]

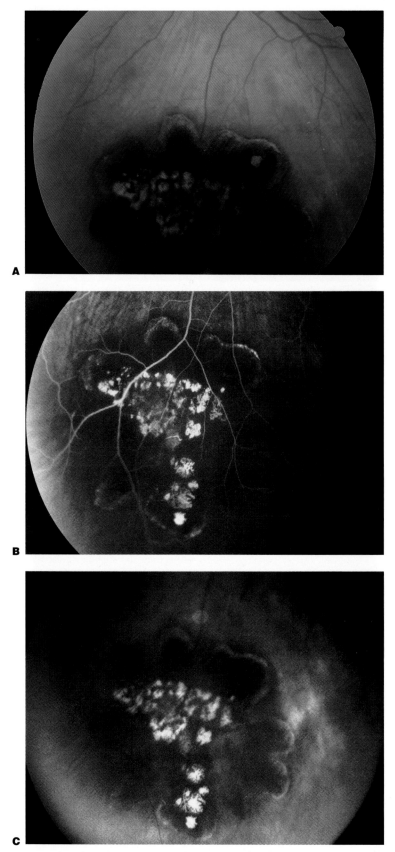

Figure 3.16 A–C Congenital Hypertrophy Of The Retinal Pigment Epithelium
Twelve years earlier, this 50 year-old female was found to have a pigmented, sharply demarcated, flat lesion (Figure 3.16A). Note the lacunae and border of depigmentation. The early fluorescein angiogram (Figure 3.16B) shows hypofluorescence of the lesion and hyperfluorescence in the areas of the lacunae. There is no late fluorescein leakage (Figure 3.16C).

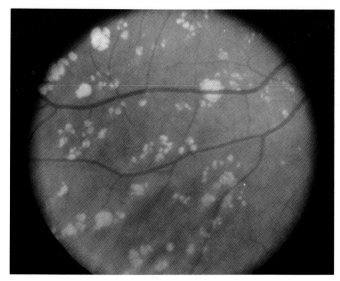

Figure 3.17 Amelanotic "Bear Tracks"
Note the multiple white lesions at the level of the retinal pigment epithelium in this asymptomatic 15 year-old female with 20/15 vision. These have been termed "polar bear tracks."

Retinal pigment epithelial adenomas and adenocarcinomas are stationary or grow slowly.[108,125] Tumors arising in the ciliary pigment epithelium may grow and encroach upon the lens, causing astigmatism, cataract, or subluxation, and the tumor may invade the anterior chamber angle.[108] A few features help differentiate an adenoma or adenocarcinoma from a malignant melanoma. More typical of an adenoma or adenocarcinoma are a dark black color and an abrupt elevation from the surrounding tissues and not a sloping margin that is more typical of a malignant melanoma.[108] Cyst formation and vitreous seeding of tumor cells is also more typical of adenoma and adenocarcinoma.[108] Fluorescein angiography and ultrasonography do not help differentiate this lesion from malignant melanoma.[80]

Combined Retina-Retinal Pigment Epithelial Hamartoma

A combined retina-retinal pigment epithelial hamartoma appears as a mass arising from the retinal pigment epithelium and retina rather than from the choroid (**Fig. 3.18,** page 50). It is believed to be congenital in origin;[38] in one large series, the diagnosis was made on average at 15 years of age.[102] It may occur anywhere in the fundus, and growth has only occasionally been documented.[33] Visual loss, however, may be progressive.[103]

A combined retina-retinal pigment epithelial hamartoma may be recognized by its three components: an epiretinal membrane, abnormal retinal vascularity within the lesion and increased pigmentation at its base. The extent of retinal vascularity[72,102] and the amount of retinal pigment epithelial proliferation can vary from lesion to lesion.[40,43,103] Most show evidence of retinal traction and vascular tortuosity due to a semitranslucent epiretinal membrane. Retinal traction seen with a combined retina-retinal pigment epithelial hamartoma is rare for a malig-

nant melanoma. Fluorescein angiography shows areas of hypofluorescence corresponding to the pigment epithelial hyperplasia; early hyperfluorescence occurs within the mass due to increased vascularity that is characteristic of this lesion.[38,40,43,103,104] The great amount of vascularity associated with a combined retina-retinal pigment epithelial hamartoma is unusual for a malignant melanoma unless a melanoma has an associated rupture of Bruch's membrane. The vessels associated with a combined retina-retinal pigment epithelial hamartoma tend to be fine, whereas tumor vessels are large. Late leakage of these fine tumor vessels seen in a combined retina-retinal pigment epithelial hamartoma is common.[38,104]

Benign Diffuse Uveal Melanocytic Proliferation

An unusual and rare pigmented lesion is benign diffuse uveal melanocytic proliferation (**Fig. 3.19A, B,** page 51) and is associated with either occult or previously diagnosed systemic malignancy.[6,45,71,97,99] Patients suffer progressive loss of vision. Early eye findings include multiple, round or oval, subtle red patches at the level of the retinal pigment epithelium. This pattern corresponds to multifocal areas of early hyperfluorescence on a fluorescein angiogram (**Fig. 3.19C–E**). Other manifestations are multiple, bilateral, pigmented choroidal nodules associated with retinal detachment. Amelanotic areas of choroidal thickening also may be seen. This appearance may be interpreted as multiple metastatic tumors. The uvea appears diffusely thickened to about 2 mm. Iris nodules, cataract, extrascleral pigmented lesions,[97] and pigmentation of the buccal mucosa may be noted (**Fig. 3.19F**).

Histologically, these eyes have a diffuse, uveal proliferation of primarily benign-appearing spindle cells and some areas of epithelioid cells.[6] However, the histologic appearance may be difficult to distinguish from a choroidal malignant melanoma.[71,97] Mitotic figures are rare and scleral infiltration may be present. Although the choriocapillaris is spared, depigmentation and degeneration of the retinal pigment epithelium occurs.[45]

CHOROIDAL OSTEOMA

Choroidal osteoma (**Fig. 3.20,** page 52) occurs most commonly in the juxtapapillary and macular area in young women.[11,43,44] Initially, it may appear orange and similar to a choroidal hemangioma.[43,123] Over time, depigmentation of the retinal pigment epithelium occurs, and the osteoma becomes more whitish-yellow.[43,44] This appearance is similar to an amelanotic melanoma or metastatic carcinoma. Choroidal osteoma is bilateral in about 20% of cases. Small, vascular "spiders" can occasionally be seen over the surface of the lesion.[11,43] Of greatest help in the diagnosis is the ultrasonographic demonstration of calcification,[11,43,44,58,63] though this can also be proved with plain x-ray or computed tomography. Magnetic resonance imaging of a choroidal osteoma demonstrates a bright T_1-weighted image and an

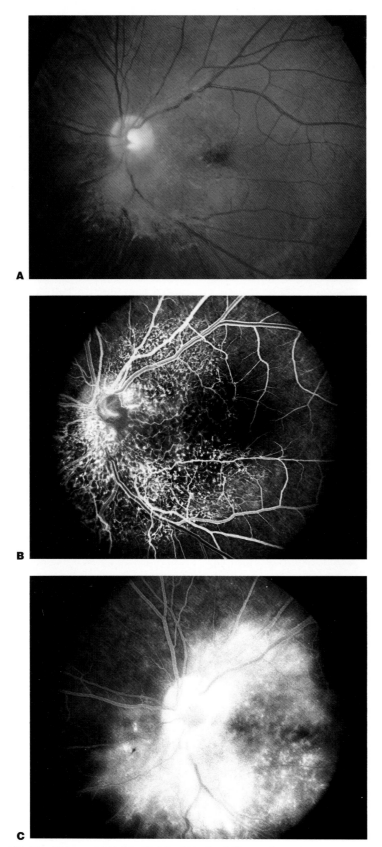

Figure 3.18 A–C Combined Retinal Pigment Epithelial And Retinal Hamartoma

Note the dilated and tortuous retinal vessels, the epiretinal membrane, and the increased pigmentation around the temporal and inferior juxtapapillary areas (Figure 3.18A). The fluorescein angiogram demonstrates these tortuous, telangiectatic vessels (Figure 3.18B) and substantial fluorescein leakage (Figure 3.18C). (Courtesy of Andrew Schachat, MD.)

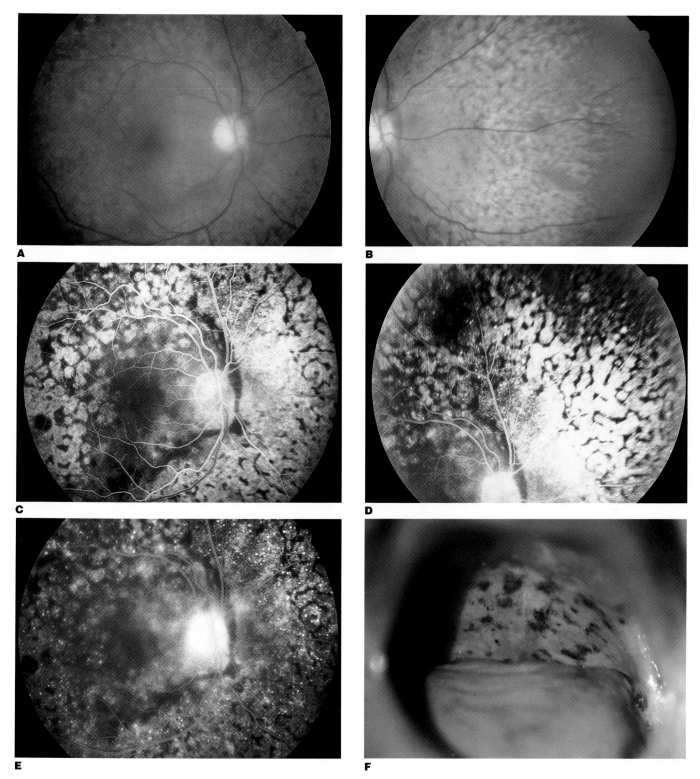

Figure 3.19 A–F Bilateral Diffuse Uveal Melanocytic Proliferation

This 62 year-old male was seen with a several month history of reduced vision in both eyes. Visual acuity was 9/200 in the right eye and 6/200 in the left eye. Note the diffuse hypo- and hyperpigmented changes of the retinal pigment epithelium (Figs. 3.19A & B). There was an extensive exudative retinal detachment in each eye with shifting fluid. The fluorescein angiogram showed many circular areas of hyperfluorescence as well as many pinpoint areas of hyperfluorescence (Figs 3.19C–E). He also had hyperpigmented patches in his buccal mucosa (Figure 3.19F). He was subsequently found to have metastatic poorly differentiated carcinoma in his chest without a known primary.

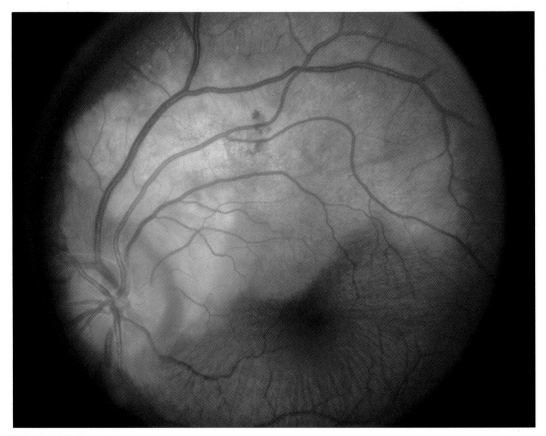

Figure 3.20 Choroidal Osteoma
This 20 year-old female had a visual acuity of 20/15 in each eye. Note the whitish-yellowish choroidal mass superotemporal to the left disc. An ultrasound examination confirmed the presence of calcification.

area of somewhat low intensity on a T_2-weighted image.[25] Use of gadolinium-DPTA as a contrast agent shows enhancement with a T_1-weighted image. The etiology of these lesions is not certain, but they can develop following inflammation and may progress or disappear or decalcify during subsequent observation[58,63,123,124] or following laser photocoagulation.

RETINAL DETACHMENT

In the past, rhegmatogenous retinal detachment was the most frequent clinical misdiagnosis among enucleated eyes that were later found to contain a malignant melanoma.[23,26,53,94,95,116] Detection of a diffuse melanoma producing a retinal detachment may be particularly difficult. Some eyes, mistakenly considered to have a rhegmatogenous retinal detachment, and not an exudative retinal detachment associated with a malignant melanoma, have undergone one or more retinal reattachment surgeries.[10] Such surgery may affect the prognosis not only because the diagnosis and treatment of malignant melanoma will be delayed, but also because surgical maneuvers (such as drainage of subretinal fluid) may promote the extraocular spread of melanoma cells.[10]

A rhegmatogenous retinal detachment is recongnized by the presence of a retinal tear, whereas an exudative retinal detachment (frequently associated with a malignant melanoma) typically has shifting fluid. Since approximately 6% of the normal population have a retinal break, the presence of a retinal break in a patient with a retinal detachment does not preclude an exudative retinal detachment caused by a malignant melanoma. Care should be taken to decide if the shape of the retinal detachment is consistent with the location of the retinal break in those instances where one is present and if the subretinal fluid shifts.

POSTERIOR SCLERITIS

The diagnosis of posterior scleritis is not easily made. Patients with posterior scleritis frequently experience pain, though some may not.[7] These patients often have a history of rheumatoid arthritis. Ophthalmoscopic examination may reveal a somewhat well-circumscribed inflammatory mass lesion that is usually the same color as the surrounding fundus **(Fig. 3.21)**.[7] Choroidal folds, retinal striae, and evidence of disc edema may be seen. These are uncommon with a malignant melanoma.[7] Dilated

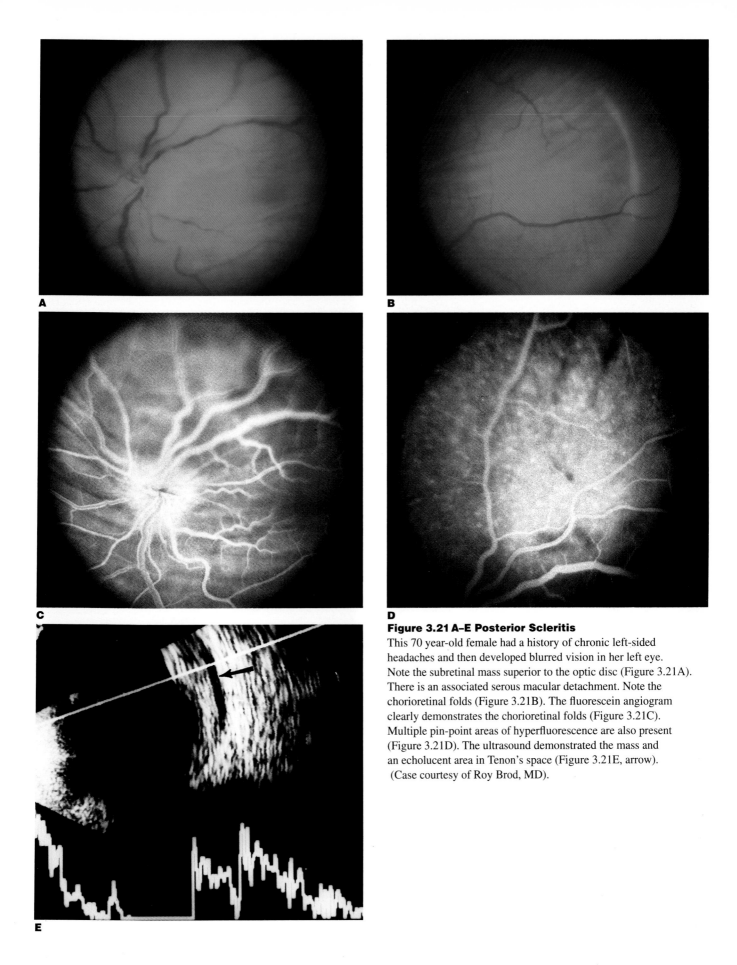

Figure 3.21 A–E Posterior Scleritis

This 70 year-old female had a history of chronic left-sided headaches and then developed blurred vision in her left eye. Note the subretinal mass superior to the optic disc (Figure 3.21A). There is an associated serous macular detachment. Note the chorioretinal folds (Figure 3.21B). The fluorescein angiogram clearly demonstrates the chorioretinal folds (Figure 3.21C). Multiple pin-point areas of hyperfluorescence are also present (Figure 3.21D). The ultrasound demonstrated the mass and an echolucent area in Tenon's space (Figure 3.21E, arrow). (Case courtesy of Roy Brod, MD).

episcleral vessels or evidence of anterior scleritis (frequently associated with posterior scleritis) should be sought during the examination. Fluorescein angiography may reveal pinpoint and larger areas of hyperfluorescence.[7] Ultrasonography usually shows high reflectivity within the retinal and choroidal layers, a thickened sclera, fluid in Tenon's space **(Fig. 3.21E)**, and, frequently, a flattened posterior pole.[7] A high degree of clinical suspicion is necessary to make this diagnosis.[7]

OTHER INFLAMMATORY CONDITIONS

Other inflammatory conditions, such as choroiditis and sarcoid granuloma, may lead to retinal detachment, focal inflammatory masses, or extensive thickening of the choroid, any of which may resemble a choroidal malignant melanoma.[94,106] The finding of nonpigmented vitreous cells is helpful. It should be noted that reactive retinal pigment epithelial hyperplasia may be associated with an inflammatory condition.[65]

RETINOSCHISIS

Retinoschisis, particularly when bullous, has led to enucleation of eyes because of suspected malignant melanoma.[26,116] This frequently bilateral condition is most commonly found inferotemporally. The retina is usually thinned, outer layer retinal holes

are frequent, and the underlying choroidal markings are easily visualized.[105] On ultrasonography, a smooth, mobile, dome-shaped structure is seen that is not solid.

RETINAL ARTERIAL MACROANEURYSM

A retinal arterial macroaneurysm may bleed under the retina or in front of the retina, or both, and produce an "hour-glass hemorrhage" **(Fig. 3.22)**.[93,104] A large subretinal hemorrhage can appear as an elevated dark mass and needs to be differentiated from a malignant melanoma. Changes in the appearance of the blood as the hemorrhage resolves (dehemoglobinization) can further alter the presentation. Frequently, a whitish or grayish circular area along the course of a retinal artery may be seen near the center of the hemorrhage. This circular area represents the wall of the macroaneurysm, which may be more easily seen with a fluorescein angiogram. Some eyes with hemorrhage from a retinal arterial macroaneurysm have been enucleated with an erroneous diagnosis of malignant melanoma.

HEMORRHAGIC AND SEROUS CHOROIDAL DETACHMENT

Hemorrhagic choroidal detachment may simulate a malignant melanoma.[83,129] Older patients have a higher risk of developing a

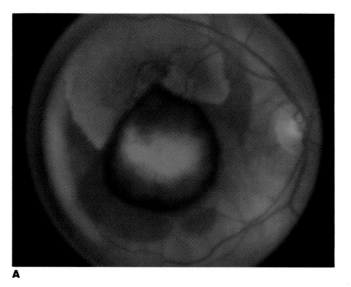
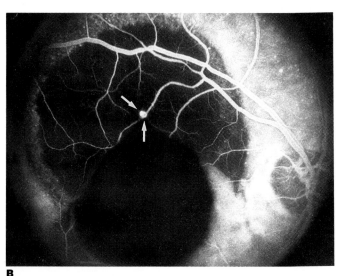

A   **B**

Figure 3.22 A & B Retinal Arterial Macroaneurysm and "Hour-Glass" Hemorrhage
This 83 year-old female developed reduced vision in her right eye 4 days earlier. The visual acuity was 4/200. Note the preretinal blood overlying the macula and the subretinal hemorrhage surrounding the macula. This is termed an "hour-glass" hemorrhage. The fluorescein angiogram shows hypofluorescence due to the hemorrhage. Note the circular area of hyperfluorescence (arrows) caused by a retinal arterial macroaneurysm just superior to the preretinal hemorrhage.

choroidal hemorrhage. Ophthalmoscopic examination may show a brownish choroidal mass. Fluorescein angiography typically shows minimal hyperfluorescence without leakage, an unusual pattern for malignant melanoma. The ultrasonographic features may be similar to a malignant melanoma, but in most cases, intrinsic tumor vascularity is not detected. Observation of these lesions shows relatively rapid resolution of the hemorrhage and therefore discretion is appropiate.

A serous choroidal detachment **(Fig. 3.23)** secondary to hypotony frequently looks like a dark choroidal mass. Choroidal folds may be present. The ultrasound clearly shows the serous, nonsolid nature of this type of choroidal elevation.

MISCELLANEOUS

Table 1.1 (page 2) lists other less commonly mistaken lesions.

SUMMARY

The differential diagnosis of malignant melanoma includes a long list of benign and malignant disorders. Care should be taken to consider all possibilities to insure an accurate diagnosis. In

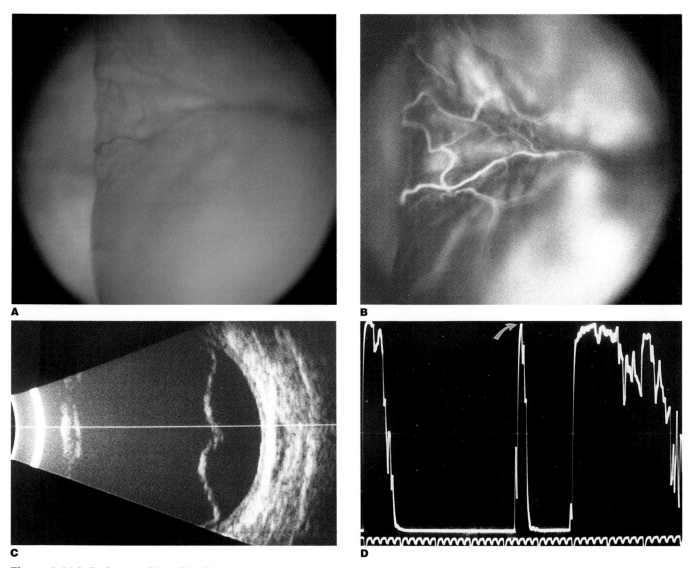

Figure 3.23 A–D Serous Choroidal Detachment
This 77 year-old female became aware of a temporal shadow in her right eye. The visual acuity was 20/30. Note the large bilobed dark choroidal mass. The fluorescein angiogram (Figure 3.23B) showed broad choroidal folds over the detachment and increased fluorescence further peripherally. Note on the B-scan ultrasound (Figure 3.23C) that the elevation appears hollow. The A-scan (Figure 3.23D) ultrasound shows a tall ultrasound peak from the retinal interface (arrow) but no echoes from within the elevation. This ultrasound pattern is typical of a serous choroidal detachment.

those cases where the presentation is atypical, observation for several weeks usually provides the most conservative means of determining the nature of a lesion if doubt exists. If the clinical situation suggests that observation is not desirable or practical, or if a period of observation has not permitted additional clues as to the diagnosis, then fine needle aspiration biopsy should be considered, and in 90% of cases will result in a diagnosis.

REFERENCES

1. Abramson DH: Computerized visual fields of choroidal melanomas. Glaucoma 10:39-48, 1988.

2. Albert DM: Ocular melanoma: a challenge to visual science. Friedenwald Lecture. Invest Ophthalmol Vis Sci 23:550-580, 1982.

3. Albert DM, Rubenstein RA, Scheie HG: Tumor metastasis to the eye. Part I. Incidence in 213 adult patients with generalized malignancy. Am J Ophthalmol 63:723-726, 1967.

4. Anand R, Augsburger JJ, Shields JA: Circumscribed choroidal hemangiomas. Arch Ophthalmol 107:1338-1342, 1989.

5. Augsburger JJ, Shields JA, Moffat KP: Circumscribed choroidal hemangiomas: Long-term visual prognosis. Retina 1:56-61, 1981.

6. Barr CC, Zimmerman LE, Curtin VT, Font RL: Bilateral diffuse melanocytic uveal tumors associated with systemic malignant neoplasms. A recently recognized syndrome. Arch Ophthalmol 100:249-255, 1982.

7. Benson WE: Posterior scleritis. Surv Ophthalmol 32:297-316, 1988.

8. Blair NP, Trempe CL: Hypertrophy of the retinal pigment epithelium associated with Gardner's syndrome. Am J Ophthalmol 90:661-667, 1980.

9. Boniuk M, Hawkins WR: Transscleral migration of pigment following cryotherapy of intraocular glioma. Tr Amer Acad Ophthalmol Oto 75:60-69, 1971.

10. Boniuk M, Zimmerman LE: Occurrence and behavior of choroidal melanomas in eyes subjected to operations for retinal detachment. Tr Amer Acad Ophthalmol Oto 66:642-658, 1962.

11. Brown GC, Shields CL: Choroidal Osteoma. In Schachat, AP (Ed): Retina. Tumors. Vol. 1. St. Louis, CV Mosby, 1989, pp 749-755.

12. Brown GC, Shields JA, Augsburger JJ: Amelanotic choroidal nevi. Ophthalmology 88:1116-1121, 1981.

13. Buettner H: Congenital hypertrophy of the retinal pigment epithelium. Am J Ophthalmol 79:177-189, 1975.

14. Buettner H: Congenital hypertrophy of the retinal pigment epithelium. In Schachat, AP (Ed): Retina. Tumors. Vol. 1. St. Louis, CV Mosby, 1989, pp 607-611.

15. Buys R, Abramson DH, Kitchin DF, et al.: Simultaneous ocular and orbital involvement from metastatic bronchogenic carcinoma. Ann Ophthalmol 14:1165-1171, 1982.

16. Byrne SF: Differential diagnosis of disciform lesions using standardized echography. In: Hillman JS, Le May MM (Eds): Ophthalmic Ultrasonography. Boston, Junk Publishers, 1983, pp 149-162.

17. Chang M, Zimmerman LE, McLean I: The persisting pseudomelanoma problem. Arch Ophthalmol 102:726-727, 1984.

18. Char DH: The management of small choroidal melanomas. Surv Ophthalmol 22:377-386, 1978.

19. Char DH: Clinical Ocular Oncology. New York, Churchill Livingstone, 1989, pp 91-149.

20. Char DH, Christensen M: Immune complexes and carcinoembryonic antigen levels in metastatic choroidal tumors. Am J Ophthalmol 89:628-631, 1980.

21. Coleman DJ, Abramson DH, Jack RL, Franzen LA: Ultrasonic diagnosis of tumors of the choroid. Arch Ophthalmol 91:344-354, 1974.

22. Cox MS: Discussion of the two preceding papers. Tr Amer Acad Ophthalmol Oto 79:307-309, 1975.

23. Davidorf FH, Letson AD, Weiss ET, Levine E: Incidence of misdiagnosed and unsuspected choroidal melanomas. A 50-year experience. Arch Ophthalmol 101:410-412, 1983.

24. De Bustros S, Augsburger JJ, Shields JA, et al.: Intraocular metastases from cutaneous malignant melanoma. Arch Ophthalmol 103:937-940, 1985.

25. DePotter P, Shields JA, Shields CL, Rao VM: Magnetic resonance imaging in choroidal osteoma. Retina 11:221-223, 1991.

26. Ferry AP: Lesions mistaken for malignant melanoma of the posterior uvea. Arch Ophthalmol 72:463-469, 1964.

27. Ferry AP, Font FL: The biologic behavior and pathological features of carcinoma metastatic to the eye and orbit. Tr Am Ophthalmol Soc 71:373-425, 1973.

28. Fine SL, Collaborative Ocular Melanoma Study Group: Second non-ocular cancers in patients with choroidal melanoma. Ophthalmology (Supp) 95:128, 1988.

29. Flindall RJ, Drance SM: Visual field studies of benign choroidal melanomata. Arch Ophthalmol 81:41-44, 1969.

30. Flindall RJ, Gass JDM: A histopathologic fluorescein angiographic correlative study of malignant melanomas of the choroid. Can J Ophthalmol 6:258-267, 1971.

31. Folberg R: Other tumors of the retinal pigment epithelium. In Schachat AP (Ed): Retina. Tumors. Vol. 1. St. Louis, CV Mosby, 1989, pp 619-621.

32. Font FL, Naumann G, Zimmerman LE: Primary malignant melanoma of the skin metastatic to the eye and orbit. Report of ten cases and review of the literature. Am J Ophthalmol 63:738-754, 1967.

33. Font RL, Moura RA, Shetlar DJ, et al.: Combined hamartoma of sensory retina and retinal pigment epithelium. Retina 9:302-311, 1989.

34. Freedman MI, Folk JC: Metastatic tumors to the eye and orbit. Patient survival and clinical characteristics. Arch Ophthalmol 105:1215-1219, 1987.

35. Fuller DG, Snyder WB, Hutton WL, Vaiser A: Ultrasonographic features of choroidal malignant melanomas. Arch Ophthalmol 97:1465-1472, 1979.

36. Ganley JP, Comstock GW: Benign nevi and malignant melanomas of the choroid. Am J Ophthalmol 76:19-25, 1973.

37. Garner A: Tumours of the retinal pigment epithelium. Br J Ophthalmol 54:715-723, 1970.

38. Gass JDM: An unusual hamartoma of the pigment epithelium and retina simulating choroidal melanoma and retinoblastoma. Tr Amer Ophthalmol Soc 71:171-185, 1973.

39. Gass JDM: Differential diagnosis of benign and malignant melanomas of the choroid. Tr Ophthalmol Soc UK 97:358-361, 1977.

40. Gass JDM: Fluorescein angiography. An aid in the differential diagnosis of intraocular tumors. Int Ophthalmol Clin 12:85-120, 1972.

41. Gass JDM: Observation of suspected choroidal and ciliary body melanomas for evidence of growth prior to enucleation. Ophthalmology 87:523-528, 1980.

42. Gass JDM: Problems in the differential diagnosis of choroidal nevi and malignant melanomas. Am J Ophthalmol 83:299-323, 1977.

43. Gass JDM: Stereoscopic Atlas of Macular Diseases. Diagnosis and Treatment. St. Louis, CV Mosby, 1987.

44. Gass JDM, Guerry RK, Jack RL, Harris G: Choroidal osteoma. Arch Ophthalmol 96:428-435, 1978.

45. Gass JDM, Gieser RG, Wilkinson CP, Beahm DE, Paultler SE: Bilateral diffuse uveal melanocytic proliferation in patients with occult carcinoma. Arch Ophthalmol 108:527-533, 1990.

46. Gitter KA, Meyer D, Sarin LK, et al.: Fluorescein and ultrasound in diagnosis of intraocular tumors. Am J Ophthalmol 66:719-730, 1968.

47. Goldberg G, Kara GB, Previte LR: The use of radioactive phosphorus (^{32}P) in the diagnosis of ocular tumors. Am J Ophthalmol 90:817-828, 1980.

48. Gonder JR, Augsburger JJ, McCarthy EF, Shields JA: Visual loss associated with choroidal nevi. Ophthalmology 89:961-965, 1982.

49. Greven CM, Slusher MM, Stanton C, Yeatts RP: Cutaneous malignant melanoma metastatic to the choroid. Arch Ophthalmol 109:547-549, 1991.

50. Haas BD, Jakobiec FA, Iwamoto T, et al.: Diffuse choroidal melanocytoma in a child. A lesion extending the spectrum of melanocytic hamartomas. Ophthalmology 93:1632-1638, 1986.

51. Hagler WS, Jarrett WH, Humphrey WT: The radioactive phosphorus uptake test in diagnosis of uveal melanoma. Arch Ophthalmol 83:548-557, 1970.

52. Hale PN, Allen RA, Straatsma BR: Benign melanomas (nevi) of the choroid and ciliary body. Arch Ophthalmol 74:532-538, 1965.

53. Harry J: Symposium on management of melanoma of the uveal tract. Errors in diagnosis. Tr Ophthalmol Soc UK 93:93-102, 1973.

54. Hayreh SS: Choroidal melanomata. Fluorescence angiographic and histopathological study. Br J Ophthalmol 54:145-160, 1970.

55. Howard GM: Erroneous clinical diagnoses of retinoblastoma and uveal melanoma. Tr Amer Acad Ophthalmol Oto 73:199-203, 1969.

56. Jampel HD, Schachat AP, Conway B, et al.: Retinal pigment hyperplasia assuming tumor-like proportions. Report of two cases. Retina 6:105-112, 1986.

57. Jensen OA: Malignant melanomas of the uvea in Denmark 1943-1952. A clinical, histopathological, and prognostic study. Acta Ophthalmol (Suppl) 75:1-220, 1963.

58. Joffe L, Shields JA, Fitzgerald JR: Osseous choristoma of the choroid. Arch Ophthalmol 96:1809-1812, 1978.

59. Joffe L, Shields JA, Osher RH, Gass JDM: Clinical and follow-up studies of melanocytomas of the optic disc. Tr Am Acad Ophthalmol Oto 86:1967-1078, 1979.

60. Joffe L, Shields JA: Melanocytoma of the optic nerve head. In Schachat AP (Ed): Retina. Tumors. Vol. 1. St. Louis, CV Mosby, 1989, vol. 1, pp 597-604.

61. Karel I, Teleska M: Fluorescence angiography in intraocular tumors. Ophthalmologica 164:161-181, 1972.

62. Karickhoff JR: Loss of visual function and visual cells in 600 cases of malignant melanoma. Am J Ophthalmol 64:268-273, 1967.

63. Katz RS, Gass JDM: Multiple choroidal osteomas developing in association with recurrent orbital inflammatory pseudotumor. Arch Ophthalmol 101:1724-1727, 1983.

64. Kindy-Degnan N, Char DH, Kroll SM: Coincident systemic malignant disease in uveal melanoma patients. Can J Ophthalmol 24:204-206, 1989.

65. Kurz GH, Zimmerman LE: Vagaries of the retinal pigment epithelium. Int Ophthalmol Clin 2:441-464, 1962.

66. Lanning R, Shields JA: Comparison of radioactive phosphorus (^{32}P) uptake test in comparable sized choroidal melanomas and hemangiomas. Am J Ophthalmol 87:769-772, 1979.

67. Lauritzen K, Augsburger JJ, Timmes J: Vitreous seeding associated with melanocytoma of the optic disc. Retina 10:60-62, 1990.

68. Letson AD, Davidorf FH: Bilateral retinal metastases from cutaneous malignant melanoma. Arch Ophthalmol 100:605-607, 1982.

69. Lewis RA, Crowder WE, Eierman LA, et al.: The Gardner syndrome. Significance of ocular features. Ophthalmology 91:916-925, 1984.

70. MacIlwaine WA, Anderson B, Klintworth GK: Enlargement of a histologically documented choroidal nevus. Am J Ophthalmol 87:480-486, 1979.

71. Margo CE, Pavan PR, Gendelman D, Gragoudas E: Bilateral melanocytic uveal tumors associated with systemic non-ocular malignancy. Retina 7:137-141, 1987.

72. McDonald HR, Abrams GW, Burke JM, Neuwirth J: Clinicopathologic results of vitreous surgery for epiretinal membranes in patients with combined retinal and retinal pigment epithelial hamartomas. Am J Ophthalmol 100:806-813, 1985.

73. McKelvey JAW, Rosen ES, Lucas DR: Photographic methods in the diagnosis of choroidal malignant melanomata. Tr Ophthalmol Soc UK 93:103-106, 1973.

74. Mewis L, Young SE: Breast carcinoma metastatic to the choroid. Analysis of 67 patients. Ophthalmology 89:147-151, 1982.

75. Meyer E, Navon D, Zonis S: The role of carcinoembryonic antigen in surveillance of patients with choroidal malignant melanoma: A prospective study. Ann Ophthalmol 19:24-25, 1987.

76. Michelson JB, Felberg NT, Shields JA, Foster L: Carcinoembryonic antigen-positive metastatic adenocarcinoma of the choroid. Arch Ophthalmol 93:794-796, 1975.

77. Michelson JB, Felberg NT, Shields JA: Carcinoembryonic antigen. Its role in the evaluation of intraocular malignant tumors. Arch Ophthalmol 94:414-416, 1976.

78. Michelson JB, Felberg NT, Shields JA: Evaluation of metastatic cancer to the eye. Carcinoembryonic antigen and gamma glutamyl transpeptidase. Arch Ophthalmol 95:692-694, 1977.

79. Mims JL, Shields JA: Follow-up studies of suspicious choroidal nevi. Tr Am Acad Ophthalmol Oto 85:929-943, 1978.

80. Minckler D, Allen AW: Adenocarcinoma of the retinal pigment epithelium. Arch Ophthalmol 96:2252-2254, 1978.

81. Minckler D, Font RL, Shields JA: Non-melanoma ocular lesions with positive ^{32}P tests. In Jakobiec F (Ed): Ocular and Adnexal Tumors. Birmingham, Aesculapius Publishers, 1978, pp 245-256.

82. Minning CA, Davidorf FH: Ossoinig's angle of ultrasonic absorption and its role in the diagnosis of malignant melanoma. Ann Ophthalmol 14:564-568, 1982.

83. Morgan CM, Gragoudas ES: Limited choroidal hemorrhage mistaken for a choroidal melanoma. Ophthalmology 94:41-46, 1987.

84. Naumann G, Yanoff M, Zimmerman LE: Histogenesis of malignant melanoma of uvea. Arch Ophthalmol 76:784-796, 1966.

85. Naumann G, Zimmerman LE, Yanoff M: Visual field defect associated with choroidal nevus. Am J Ophthalmol 62:914-917, 1966.

86. Naumann GOH, Hellner K, Naumann LR: Pigmented nevi of the choroid. Clinical study of secondary changes in the overlying tissues. Tr Am Acad Ophthalmol Oto 75:110-123, 1971.

87. Norton EWD, Gutman F: Fluorescein angiography and hemangiomas of the choroid. Arch Ophthalmol 78:121-125, 1967.

88. Oosterhuis JA, de Wolf-Rouendaal D: Differential diagnosis of very small melanomas and naevi of the choroid. In Oosterhuis JA (Ed): Ophthalmic Tumors. Dordrecht, Junk Publishers, 1985, pp 1-8.

89. Oosterhuis JA, Pauwels EKJ, de Wolff-Rouendaal D, et al.: ^{32}Phosphorus uptake test in choroidal melanomas, naevi and haemangiomas. Doc Ophthalmol 50:9-19, 1980.

90. Ossoinig KC, Blodi FC: Preoperative differential diagnosis of tumors with echography: III. Diagnosis of intraocular tumors. In Blodi FC (Ed): Current Concepts in Ophthalmology. Vol. 4. St. Louis, CV Mosby, 1974, pp 296-313.

91. Pettit TH, Barton A, Foos RY, Christensen RE: Fluorescein angiography of choroidal melanomas. Arch Ophthalmol 83:27-38, 1970.

92. Pro M, Shields JA, Tomer TL: Serous detachment of the macula associated with presumed choroidal nevi. Arch Ophthalmol 96:1374-1377, 1978.

93. Rabb MF, Gagliano DA, Teske MP: Retinal arterial macroaneurysms. Surv Ophthalmol 33:73-96, 1988.

94. Reese AB: Pigmented tumors. In: Tumors of the Eye. Third Ed. New York, Harper & Row, 1976, pp 173-226.

95. Reese AB, Jones IS: The differential diagnosis of malignant melanoma of the choroid. Arch Ophthalmol 58:477-482, 1957.

96. Robertson DM, Campbell RJ: Errors in the diagnosis of malignant melanoma of the choroid. Am J Ophthalmol 87:269-275, 1979.

97. Rohrbach JM, Roggendorf W, Thanos S, et al.: Simultaneous bilateral diffuse melanocytic uveal hyperplasia. Am J Ophthalmol 110:49-56, 1990.

98. Rose SJ, Burke JF, Brockhurst RJ: Argon laser photoablation of a choroidal osteoma. Retina 11:224-228, 1991.

99. Ryll DL, Campbell RJ, Robertson DM, Brubaker SJ: Pseudometastatic lesions of the choroid. Ophthalmology 87:1181-1186, 1980.

100. Sahel JA, Albert DM: Choroidal nevi. In Schachat AP (Ed): Retina. Tumors. Vol. 1. St. Louis, CV Mosby, 1989, pp 625-637.

101. Sanborn GE: Choroidal hemangioma. In Schachat AP (Ed): Retina. Tumors. Vol. 1. St. Louis, CV Mosby, 1989, pp 757-766.

102. Schachat AP, Shields JA, Fine SL, et al.: Combined hamartomas of the retina and retinal pigment epithelium. Ophthalmology 91:1609-1615, 1984.

103. Schachat AP: Combined hamartoma of the retina and retinal pigment epithelium. In Schachat AP (Ed): Retina. Tumors. Vol. 1. St. Louis, CV Mosby, 1989, pp 613-617.

104. Schatz H, Burton TC, Yannuzzi LA, Rabb M: Interpretation of Fundus Fluorescein Angiography. St. Louis, CV Mosby, 1978.

105. Shields JA: Current approaches to the diagnosis and management of choroidal melanomas. Surv Ophthalmol 21:443-463, 1977.

106. Shields JA: The differential diagnosis of malignant melanoma of the choroid. In Peyman GA, Apple DJ, Sanders DR (Eds): Intraocular Tumors. New York, Appleton-Century-Crofts, 1977, pp 1-8.

107. Shields JA: Accuracy and limitations of the ^{32}P test in the diagnosis of ocular tumors: An analysis of 500 cases. Tr Am Acad Ophthalmol Oto 85:950-966, 1978.

108. Shields JA: Diagnosis and Management of Intraocular Tumors. St. Louis, CV Mosby, 1983.

109. Shields JA, Augsburger JJ, Bernardino V, et al.: Melanocytoma of the ciliary body and iris. Am J Ophthalmol 89:632-635, 1980.

110. Shields JA, Augsburger JJ, Brown GC, Stephens RF: The differential diagnosis of posterior uveal melanoma. Ophthalmology 87:518-522, 1980.

111. Shields JA, Font RL: Melanocytoma of the choroid clinically simulating a malignant melanoma. Arch Ophthalmol 87:396-400, 1972.

112. Shields JA, Green WR, McDonald PR: Uveal pseudomelanoma due to posttraumatic pigmentary migration. Arch Ophthalmol 89:519-522, 1973.

113. Shields JA, McDonald PR: Improvements in the diagnosis of posterior uveal melanomas. Arch Ophthalmol 91:259-264, 1974.

114. Shields JA, Shields CL, Eagle RC, et al.: Malignant melanoma associated with melanocytoma of the optic disc. Ophthalmol 97:225-230, 1990.

115. Shields JA, Tasman WS: B-Scan ultrasonography of lesions simulating choroidal melanomas. Mod Probl Ophthalmol 18:57-63, 1977.

116. Shields JA, Zimmerman LE: Lesions simulating malignant melanoma of the posterior uvea. Arch Ophthalmol 89:466-471, 1973.

117. Smith LT, Irvine AR: Diagnostic significance of orange pigment accumulation over choroidal tumors. Am J Ophthalmol 76:212-216, 1973.

118. Spiers F, Jensen OA: Pseudo-epitheliomatous hyperplasia of the retinal pigment epithelium. Acta Ophthalmol 41:722-727, 1963.

119. Stephens RF, Shields JA: Diagnosis and management of cancer metastatic to the uvea: A study of 70 cases. Ophthalmology 86:1336-1349, 1979.

120. Stow NM: Hyperplasia of the pigment epithelium of the retina simulating a neoplasm. Tr Am Acad Ophthalmol Oto 53:674-677, 1949.

121. Tamler E: A clinical study of choroidal nevi. A follow-up report. Arch Ophthalmol 84:29-32, 1970.

122. Tamler E, Maumenee AE: A clinical study of choroidal nevi. Arch Ophthalmol 62:196-202, 1959.

123. Trimble SN, Schatz H: Choroidal osteoma after intraocular inflammation. Am J Ophthalmol 96:759-764, 1983.

124. Trimble SN, Schatz H: Decalcification of a choroidal osteoma. Br J Ophthalmol 75:61-63, 1991.

125. Tso MOM, Albert DM: Pathological condition of the retinal pigment epithelium. Neoplasms and nodular non-neoplastic lesions. Arch Ophthalmol 88:27-38, 1972.

126. Van Dijk RA: The ^{32}P test and other methods in the diagnosis of intraocular tumors. (Thesis). Doc Ophthalmol 16:1-132, 1978.

127. Vogel MH, Zimmerman LE, Gass JDM: Proliferation of the juxtapapillary retinal pigment epithelium simulating malignant melanoma. Doc Ophthalmol 26:461-481, 1969.

128. Wharam MD, Schachat AP: Choroidal metastasis. In Schachat AP(Ed): Retina. Tumors. Vol. 1. St. Louis, CV Mosby, 1989, 739-748.

129. Williams DF, Mieler WF, Lewandowski M: Resolution of an apparent choroidal melanoma. Retina 9:131-135, 1989.

130. Witschel H, Font RL: Hemangioma of the choroid. A clinico-pathologic study of 71 cases and a review of the literature. Surv Ophthalmol 20:415-431, 1976.

131. Zimmerman LE, Garron LK: Melanocytoma of the optic disc. Int Ophthalmol Clin 2:431-440, 1962.

CHAPTER 4

HISTOPATHOLOGY

In 1931, Callender proposed a new classification system for ciliochoroidal melanomas based on cytologic characteristics. Five categories were described: spindle subtype A, spindle subtype B, fascicular, mixed, and epithelioid cell. Modifications have been made, but the classification remains very useful.

CALLENDER CLASSIFICATION

Spindle cell tumors have sheets, or whorls, of spindle-shaped cells with long, oval nuclei. Spindle subtypes are differentiated by nuclear characteristics. Subtype A cells have smaller, more slender nuclei with a delicate reticular structure and ill-defined or absent nucleoli. A longitudinal fold in the nuclear membrane is sometimes seen extending the length of the nucleus. Mitotic figures are rare or absent. Subtype B cells **(Fig. 4.1)** have a larger nucleus and a more defined nucleolus usually centrally located amid a coarser nuclear network. Mitotic figures are more common. Epithelioid cells **(Fig. 4.2)** are polygonal and larger, but Callender's original description described variability in size and shape. The nuclei are large, round or oval, and the nucleolus is distinct; sometimes two nucleoli are present. The histologic features of epithelioid cells are the most malignant and usually have the most mitotic figures. Fascicular type tumors have a pallisading arrangement of the cells and contain cells that closely

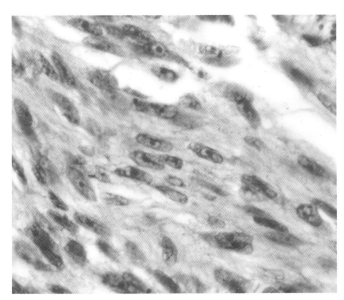

Figure 4.1 Spindle B Cell Melanoma
Note the thin cells with oval-shaped nuclei within this spindle B cell melanoma.

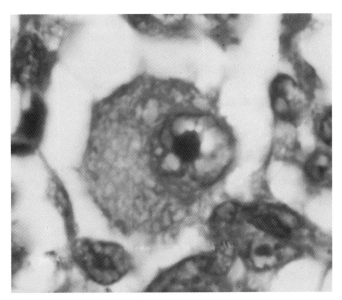

Figure 4.2 Epithelioid Cell Melanoma
Note the large round cell with a round nucleus and prominent nucleoli.

resemble spindle subtype B cells. The most common type in Callender's original report was the mixed-cell tumor. A mixed-cell tumor has an irregular mixture of spindle and epithelioid cells and occasional fascicular areas are present.

Significant for the Callender classification is the ability to provide prognostic information; spindle cell tumors have the best prognosis, and epithelioid and mixed-cell tumors have the worst prognosis (Table 8.1, page 84). Several years after Callender reported the original classification, a sixth subgroup was added. This group, termed necrotic, applies to tumors with more than 50% necrosis.[73]

The Callender classification has been critically examined.[35,37,45,49,51,57,63] Some criticisms include that the classification did not set forth guidelines indicating the proportions of cell types within each subtype group[45]. This lack of guidelines results in variability among pathologists in tumor cell-type classification; pathologists may differ when classifying the same tumor.[32,35,37,57]

The Callender classification, as with all cytologic classifications, cannot definitively classify a tumor's malignant potential.[35] Callender, in his original report of melanomas, did not have information concerning growth prior to enucleation. It has been reasoned that Callender studied melanocytic lesions with variable growth potential and, therefore, the Callender classification cannot provide a measure of biologic activity. Moreover, since none of the spindle A cell melanomas in Callender's original series were associated with metastatic death, classifying these as a malignant melanoma was probably not accurate.[35,80] The histologic features shared by spindle cell A melanomas and choroidal nevi can make differentiation impossible, and underscores the potential inaccuracy of classifying a spindle cell A tumor as a malignant melanoma or a benign nevus.

The spindle subtype A group has been reevaluated and more precise classification guidelines have been outlined.[49] Spindle cell nevi consist of spindle A cells as described above, have absent mitotic activity, and are less than 10 mm in diameter or 3 mm in elevation. Although spindle cell melanomas could be of a size similar to spindle cell nevi, cytologically, spindle cell melanomas have more atypical spindle cells. These atypical spindle cells have an increased nuclear-to-cytoplasmic ratio, clumped chromatin, and distinct nucleoli. A combined spindle A and B type melanoma, simply designated spindle cell melanoma, was proposed.

Other modifications of the Callender classification have been suggested. The fascicular group is no longer used at the Armed Forces Institute of Pathology. Instead, classification of these tumors is according to cytologic characteristics and not according to the general cellular arrangement.[80]

The variability in size of epithelioid cells has been evaluated. An epithelioid cell can be smaller with less cytoplasm and a smaller nucleus than the classic Callender epithelioid cell but still possess a large eosinophilic nucleoli. Moreover, these smaller epithelioid cells are less cohesive as are classic epithelioid cells.[47,48] This modification resulted in the reclassification of many spindle B type tumors as mixed-cell type. This modified classification system produced a better correlation between prognosis for survival and histologic classification.

Computerized methods of measuring nucleolar area have been developed in an effort for more objectivity.[31,33] Prognosis for survival correlates well with the inverse standard deviation of the nucleolar area.

ASSOCIATED HISTOLOGIC FINDINGS

Benign-appearing nevus cells are frequently found at the base or along an edge of a melanoma.[4,58,77] Because of this observation, some authors speculate that most, if not all, melanomas arise from nevi,[4,76,77] but there is not complete agreement. Some series have found associated nevus cells less frequently.[5] Also, nevus-like structures can occur at the base of a metastatic lesion,[1] and in relation to experimentally implanted choroidal tumors.[2] Moreover, an interesting report documented a malignant melanoma arising in an area of the choroid (de novo) that previously did not contain an ophthalmoscopically visible nevus.[62]

A review of these reports suggests that it is likely that melanomas arise not only de novo but also from pre-existing nevi and melanosis.[3] Because nevi are much more frequent than malignant melanoma, transformation is infrequent. A nevus may transform into a malignant melanoma,[68] although this event has been estimated to occur only once for every 5,000 choroidal nevi per year.[34]

Growth of a melanoma and an increase in height may produce a break in Bruch's membrane and an overlying projection through Bruch's membrane ("collar-button") into the subretinal space (**Fig. 4.3**).[11,37,58,65,80] Extension into the subretinal space or tumor infiltration of the retina and extension into the vitreous space may occasionally produce shedding of melanoma cells and, rarely, distal subretinal or preretinal tumor foci.[58,69,80] Pigment-laden macrophages, or melanoma cells, may disperse throughout the vitreous and anterior chamber and may lodge within the trabecular meshwork, producing obstruction and melanomalytic glaucoma.[24,50,59,71,75] This is typically associated with ciliary body tumors and tumor necrosis. There is histologic evidence of rubeosis in 9% to 15% of melanomas and is more common in diffuse and necrotic tumors.[7,10,29,70]

A diffuse pattern of growth occurs in approximately 5% of malignant melanomas.[29,60] A diffuse malignant melanoma produces extraocular extension in 40% to 53% of cases (two-thirds of which are multiple extensions) and has a worse prognosis.

A little scleral extension, either through a scleral channel or by direct scleral infiltration, is common, and occurs microscopically in 23% to 80% of cases;[5,20–22,37,41,46,53,58,64] serial tumor sectioning results in the highest rate of detection.[21,22] Extraocular extension can occur with infiltration along the scleral canals of

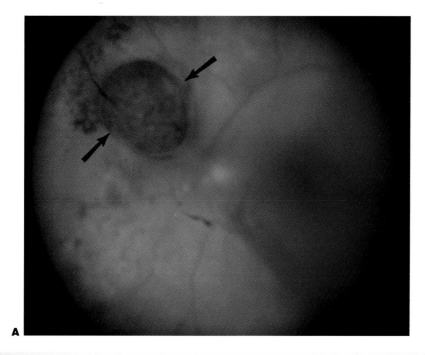

A

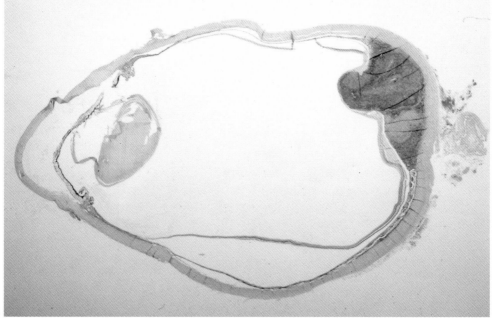

B

Figure 4.3 A & B Collar-Button Malignant Melanoma

This 64 year-old female had a 10 mm × 12 mm peripapillary choroidal melanoma that was 4.9 mm thick. Note the collar-button configuration (Figure 4.3A, arrows). The area of the melanoma that has broken through Bruch's membrane and produced the collar-button configuration can be seen histologically (Figure 4.3B).

ciliary vessels and nerves (**Fig. 4.4**) and along the vortex vessels (**Fig. 4.5**).[5,80] Direct extension within ciliary nerves can also occur.[27,74] When tumor invades a choroidal vessel, tumor growth may extend within the vessel lumen and into a vortex vein.[5,80] Less commonly, spontaneous scleral necrosis (associated with larger, more necrotic tumors and panophthalmitis), or iatrogenic scleral necrosis (as a complication of plaque radiotherapy or retinal detachment surgery), may permit extraocular tumor extension.[7,58,80] Juxtapapillary tumors may extend through the optic nerve, presumably because Bruch's membrane resistance is less along the disc edge where Bruch's membrane terminates.[80] Intracranial spread via this pathway is rare.[58]

Balloon cells associated with malignant melanomas are large pale cells occasionally found among melanoma cells and represent only a descriptive term without prognostic significance.[6,40,61] They are more common near the base or periphery of the tumor and develop possibly because of defective premelanosome synthesis or lipid deposition.[6,36,40,61,80]

Lymphocytic infiltration can occur at the base of a melanoma in the absence of tumor necrosis, or it may be associated with tumor vessels. Lymphocytic infiltration rarely occurs within noninvolved uvea.[18] Correlation between the extent of lymphocytic infiltration and prognosis for survival has not been proven.[18]

Histologic examination shows tumor necrosis in 4% to 27% of cases.[6,7,9,17,37,54,59] Tumor necrosis may alter clinical findings and result in erroneous and delayed diagnosis.[7,44,59] Two kinds of necrosis have been delineated. The first, a diffuse lytic and cellular necrosis, was associated with varying degrees of cell necrosis, cystic spaces, dispersed pigment-laden macrophages, inflammation, and inflammatory chorioretinal adhesions. The second variety, coagulation necrosis, had a sharply demarcated infarct area and inflammatory cells infiltrated the entire tumor.

The pathogenesis of tumor necrosis is not certain. An immunological response producing tumor regression has been suggested.[59] Humoral and cellular immune activity occur with malignant melanoma,[14,16,23,25,26,52,55,56] but how this correlates with prognosis and tumor regression is not clear. A complete review of the immunologic factors associated with malignant melanomas and tumors has been addressed by others.[11–13,15,19,38] Other factors associated with tumor necrosis may include ischemia due to the tumor outgrowing its blood supply[24] or occlusion induced by neoplastic vascular invasion.[78]

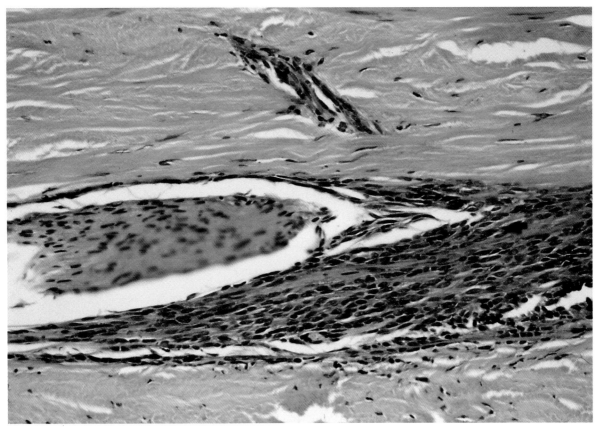

Figure 4.4 Malignant Melanoma And Intrascleral Tumor Extension
Note the extension of melanoma cells along the ciliary nerve.

Cavitation or cyst formation within malignant melanoma occurs infrequently and, as with tumor necrosis, may cause diagnostic difficulty. One such case demonstrated both cystic and solid ophthalmoscopic and ultrasonographic findings.[79] Histologically, multiple cavities without necrosis were present. Although previously assumed to be the result of tumor necrosis,[58] the pathogenesis is not known.

Alterations of the retina overlying a malignant melanoma may include microcystoid degeneration, loss of photoreceptors, and retinal pigment epithelial proliferation or degeneration.[39,42,58,72,80] Mechanisms may include tumor compression and loss of blood supply by obliteration of the choriocapillaris overlying the tumor, or perhaps a toxic effect of metabolites.[39,80] In more intact areas of the retinal pigment epithelium, drusen can be noted, and areas of lipofuscin (orange pigment) accumulation within retinal pigment epithelial cells or macrophages.[5,28,30,66,67] Subretinal neovascularization also may develop. Degenerative changes in the inner retinal layers may occur, and can explain visual field defects that are larger than the tumor.[39,80] Secondary retinal detachment is a frequent finding, as is migration of subretinal pigment cells;[5,39,42,43,58,80] accumulation of these pigment cells usually occurs at the borders of the retinal detachment.[43,58]

SUMMARY

Although imperfect, the Callender classification represents a hallmark in the history of malignant melanoma studies and provides important information to estimate the prognosis for survival for a given tumor. A more objective method includes calculation of the inverse standard deviation of the nucleolar area. Another important histologic finding that influences the prognosis for survival is the presence or absence of extraocular tumor extension. Growth of the tumor and tumor necrosis may produce other associated histologic alterations.

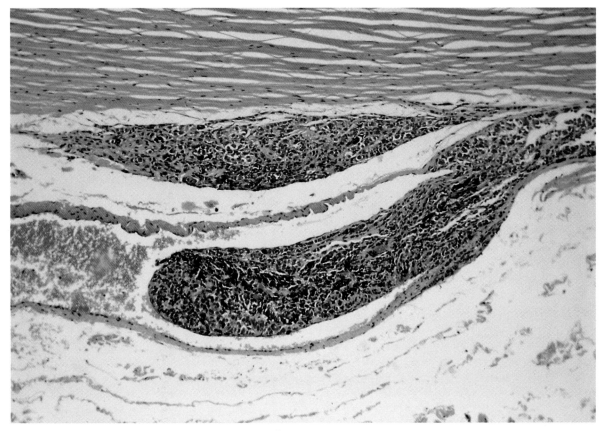

Figure 4.5 Malignant Melanoma and Extrascleral Tumor Extension
Note the extension of the melanoma along the lumen of the vortex vein.

REFERENCES

1. Albert DM, Gaasterland DE, Caldwell JBH, et al.: Bilateral metastatic choroidal melanoma, nevi, and cavernous degeneration. Arch Ophthalmol 87:39-47, 1972.

2. Albert DM, Lahav M, Packer S, Yimoyines D: Histogenesis of malignant melanomas of the uvea. Occurrence of nevus-like structures in experimental choroidal tumors. Arch Ophthalmol 92:318-323, 1974.

3. Albert DM: Ocular melanoma: A challenge to visual science. Friedenwald Lecture. Invest Ophthalmol Vis Sci 23:550-580, 1982.

4. Arnesen K, Nornes M: Malignant melanoma of the choroid as related to coexistent benign nevus. Acta Ophthalmol 53:139-152, 1975.

5. Barry DR: Malignant melanoma of the choroid. A review of the histopathology of 100 cases. Trans Ophthalmol Soc UK 93:647-664, 1973.

6. Blodi FC: Pathology of choroidal melanomas. Unusual aspects confusing the clinical diagnosis. Trans Ophthalmol Soc UK 97:362-367, 1977.

7. Bujara K: Necrotic malignant melanomas of the choroid and ciliary body. A clinicopathological and statistical study. Graefes Arch Klin Exp Ophthalmol 219:40-43, 1982.

8. Callender GR: Malignant melanotic tumors of the eye: A study of histologic types in 111 cases. Tr Am Acad Ophthalmol Oto 36:131-142, 1931.

9. Callender GR, Wilder HC, Ash JE: Five hundred melanomas of the choroid and ciliary body followed five years or longer. Am J Ophthalmol 25:962-967, 1942.

10. Cappin JM: Malignant melanoma and rubeosis iridis. Histopathological and statistical study. Br J Ophthalmol 57:815-824, 1973.

11. Char DH: Clinical Ocular Oncology. New York, Churchill Livingstone, 1989, pp 91-149.

12. Char DH: Immunologic aspects and management of malignant intraocular pigmented neoplasms. In Peyman GA, Apple DJ, Sanders DR (Eds): Intraocular Tumors. New York, Appleton/Century/Crofts, 1977, pp 87-103.

13. Char DH: Immunologic mechanisms in choroidal melanoma. Tr Ophthalmol Soc UK 97:389-393, 1977.

14. Char DH: Inhibition of leukocyte migration with melanoma associated antigens in choroidal tumors. Invest Ophthalmol 16:176-179, 1977.

15. Char DH: Immunology of Uveitis and Ocular Tumors. New York, Grune & Stratton, 1978, pp 74-109.

16. Char DH, Hollinshead A, Cogan DG, et al.: Cutaneous delayed hypersensitivity reactions to soluble melanoma antigen in patients with ocular malignant melanoma. New Engl J Med 291:274-277, 1974.

17. Char DH, Howes EL, Fries PD, et al.: Uveal melanoma with opaque media: Absence of definitive diagnosis before enucleation. Can J Ophthalmol 23:22-26, 1988.

18. Davidorf FH, Lang JR: Lymphocytic infiltration in choroidal melanoma and its prognostic significance. Trans Ophthalmol Soc UK 97:394-401, 1977.

19. Davidorf FH, Lang JR: Immunology and immunotherapy of malignant uveal melanomas. In Peyman GA, Apple DJ, Sanders DR (Eds): Intraocular Tumors. New York, Appleton/Century/Crofts, 1977, pp 119-133.

20. Davies WS: Malignant melanomas of the choroid and ciliary body. A clinicopathologic study. Am J Ophthalmol 55:541-546, 1963.

21. De Wolff-Rouendaal D, Oosterhuis JA: Histology of small melanomas. Doc Ophthalmol 50:21-26, 1980.

22. Donders PC: Malignant melanoma of the choroid. Trans Ophthalmol Soc UK 93:745-751, 1973.

23. Donoso LA, Augsburger JJ, Shields JA, et al.: Metastatic uveal melanoma. Correlation between survival time and cytomorphometry of primary tumors. Arch Ophthalmol 104:76-78, 1986.

24. El Baba F, Hagler WS, De La Cruz A, Green WR: Choroidal melanoma with pigment dispersion in vitreous and melanomalytic glaucoma. Ophthalmology 95:370-377, 1988.

25. Federman JL, Clark WH: Circulating antibodies in patients with intraocular melanomas. In Peyman GA, Apple DJ, Sanders DR (Eds): Intraocular Tumors. New York, Appleton/Century/Croft, 1977, pp 105-111.

26. Federman JL, Felberg NT, Shields JA: Effect of local treatment on antibody levels in malignant melanoma of the choroid. Tr Ophthalmol Soc UK 97:436-439, 1977.

27. Ferry AP: Orbital extension of choroidal melanoma within a short posterior ciliary nerve. Am J Ophthalmol 98:517-518, 1984.

28. Fishman GA, Apple DJ, Goldberg MF: Retinal and pigment epithelial alterations over choroidal malignant melanomas. Ann Ophthalmol 7:487-492, 1975.

29. Font RL, Spaulding AG, Zimmerman LE: Diffuse malignant melanoma of the uveal tract: A clinicopathologic report of 54 cases. Tr Amer Acad Ophthalmol Oto 72:877-894, 1968.

30. Font RL, Zimmerman LE, Armaly MF: The nature of the orange pigment over a choroidal melanoma. Histochemical and electron microscopical observations. Arch Ophthalmol 91:359-362, 1974.

31. Gamel JW, McLean IW: Modern developments in histopathologic assessment of uveal melanomas. Ophthalmology 91:679-684, 1984.

32. Gamel JW, McLean IW: Quantitative analysis of the Callender classification of uveal melanoma cells. Arch Ophthalmol 95:686-691, 1977.

33. Gamel JW, McLean I, Greenberg RA, et al.: Objective assessment of the malignant potential of intraocular melanomas with standard microslides stained with hematoxylin-eosin. Hum Pathol 16:689-692, 1985.

34. Ganley JP, Comstock GW: Benign nevi and malignant melanomas of the choroid. Am J Ophthalmol 76:19-25, 1973.

35. Gass JDM: Problems in the differential diagnosis of choroidal nevi and malignant melanomas. Am J Ophthalmol 83:299-323, 1977.

36. Jakobiec FA, Shields JA, Desjardins L, Iwamoto T: Balloon cell melanomas of the ciliary body. Arch Ophthalmol 97:1667-1692, 1979.

37. Jensen OA: Malignant melanomas of the uvea in Denmark 1943-1952. A clinical, histopathological, and prognostic study. Acta Ophthalmol (Suppl) 75:1-220, 1963.

38. Kaplan HJ: Lymphocyte subpopulations in uveal malignant melanoma. Am J Ophthalmol 101:483-485, 1986.

39. Karickhoff JR: Loss of visual function and visual cells in 600 cases of malignant melanoma. Am J Ophthalmol 64:268-273, 1967.

40. Khalil MK: Balloon cell malignant melanoma of the choroid: Ultrastructural studies. Br J Ophthalmol 67:579-584, 1983.

41. Kidd MN, Lyness RW, Patterson CC, et al.: Prognostic factors in malignant melanoma of the choroid: A retrospective survey of cases occurring in Northern Ireland between 1965-1980. Trans Ophthalmol Soc UK 105:114-121, 1986.

42. Kirk HO, Petty RW: Malignant melanoma of the choroid. A correlation of clinical and histological findings. Arch Ophthalmol 56:843-860, 1956.

43. Lahav M, Gutman I: Subretinal pigment cells in malignant melanoma of the choroid. Am J Ophthalmol 86:239-244, 1978.

44. Latkovic Z: On our cases of necrotic choroidal melanoma. In Lommatzsch PK and Blodi FC (Eds): Intraocular Tumors. New York, Springer-Verlag, 1983, pp 75-79.

45. MacRae A: Prognosis in malignant melanoma of choroid and ciliary body. Tr Ophthalmol Soc UK 73:3-30, 1953.

46. McLean IW, Foster WD, Zimmerman LE: Prognostic factors in small malignant melanomas of the choroid and ciliary body. Arch Ophthalmol 95:48-58, 1977.

47. McLean IW, Foster WD, Zimmerman LE, Gamel JW: Modification of Callender's classification of uveal melanoma at the Armed Forces Institute of Pathology. Am J Ophthalmol 96:502-509, 1983.

48. McLean IW, Foster WD, Zimmerman LE: Uveal melanoma: Location, size, cell type, and enucleation as risk factors in metastasis. Hum Pathol 13:123-132, 1982.

49. McLean IW, Zimmerman LE, Evans RM: Reappraisal of Callender's spindle A type of malignant melanoma of choroid and ciliary body. Am J Ophthalmol 86:557-564, 1978.

50. McMenamin PG, Lee WR: Ultrastructural pathology of melanomalytic glaucoma. Br J Ophthalmol 70:895-906, 1986.

51. Morgan G: The history and natural history of malignant melanomata of the uvea. Tr Ophthalmol Soc UK 93:71-78, 1973.

52. Noor MS, Rahi AHS, Morgan G, Holborow EJ: Lymphoproliferative response as an index of cellular immunity in malignant melanoma of the uvea and its correlation with the histological features of the tumour. Br J Ophthalmol 64:576-590, 1980.

53. Oosterhuis JA, de Wolf-Rouendaal D: Differential diagnosis of very small melanomas and naevi of the choroid. In Oosterhuis JA (Ed): Ophthalmic Tumors. Dordrecht, Junk Publishers, 1985, pp 1-8.

54. Paul V, Parnell L, Fraker M: Prognosis of malignant melanomas of the choroid and ciliary body. Int Ophthalmol Clin 2:387-402, 1962.

55. Priluck IA, Robertson DM, Pritchard DJ, Ilstrup DM: Immune responsiveness in patients with choroidal malignant melanoma. Am J Ophthalmol 87:215-220, 1979.

56. Rahi AHS: Immunological aspects of malignant melanoma of the choroid. Tr Ophthalmol Soc UK 93:79-91, 1973.

57. Raivio I: Uveal melanoma in Finland. An epidemiological, clinical, histological and prognostic study. Acta Ophthalmol 133:5-64, 1977.

58. Reese AB: Pigmented tumors. In Tumors of the Eye. Third Ed. New York, Harper & Row, 1976, pp 173-226.

59. Reese AB, Archila EA, Jones IS, Cooper WC: Necrosis of malignant melanomas of the choroid. Am J Ophthalmol 99:104, 1970.

60. Reese AB, Howard GM: Flat uveal melanomas. Am J Ophthalmol 64:1021-1028, 1967.

61. Riley FC: Balloon cell melanoma of the choroid. Arch Ophthalmol 92:131-133, 1974.

62. Sahel JA, Pesavento R, Frederick AR, et al.: Melanoma arising de novo over a 16-month period. Arch Ophthalmol 106:381-385, 1988.

63. Seddon JM, Polivogianis L, Hseih CC, et al.: Death from uveal melanoma. Number of epithelioid cells and inverse SD of nucleolar area as prognostic factors. Arch Ophthalmol 105:801-806, 1987.

64. Shammas H, Blodi FC: Prognostic factors in choroidal and ciliary body melanomas. Arch Ophthalmol 95:63-69, 1977.

65. Shields JA: Diagnosis and Management of Intraocular Tumors. St. Louis, CV Mosby, 1983.

66. Shields JA, Rodrigues MM, Sarin LK, et al.: Lipofuscin pigment over benign and malignant choroidal tumors. Trans Am Acad Ophthalmol Oto 81:871-881, 1976.

67. Smith LT, Irvine AR: Diagnostic significance of orange pigment accumulation over choroidal tumors. Am J Ophthalmol 76:212-216, 1973.

68. Smolin G: Malignant change of a benign melanoma. Am J Ophthalmol 61:174-177, 1966.

69. Spencer WH: Optic nerve extension of intraocular neoplasms. Am J Ophthalmol 80:465-471, 1975.

70. Terry TL, Johns JP: Uveal sarcoma-malignant melanoma. A statistical study of ninety-four cases. Am J Ophthalmol 18:903-913, 1935.

71. Van Buskirk E, Leure-du Pree AE: Pathophysiology and electron microscopy of melanomalytic glaucoma. Am J Ophthalmol 85:160-166, 1978.

72. Wallow IHL, Tso MOM: Proliferation of the retinal pigment epithelium over malignant choroidal tumors. A light and electron microscopic study. Am J Ophthalmol 73:914-926, 1972.

73. Wilder HC, Callender GR: Malignant melanoma of the choroid. Further studies on prognosis by histologic type and fiber content. Am J Ophthalmol 22:851-855, 1939.

74. Wolter JR: Orbital extension of choroidal melanoma: Within a long posterior ciliary nerve. Tr Am Ophthalmol Soc 81:47-63, 1983.

75. Yanoff M, Scheie HG: Melanomalytic glaucoma. Report of a case. Arch Ophthalmol 84:471-473, 1970.

76. Yanoff M, Zimmerman LE: Histogenesis of malignant melanomas of the uvea. II. Relationship of uveal nevi to malignant melanomas. Cancer 20:493-507, 1967.

77. Yanoff M, Zimmerman LE: Histogenesis of malignant melanomas of the uvea. III. The relationship of congenital ocular melanocytosis and neurofibromatosis to uveal melanomas. Arch Ophthalmol 77:331-336, 1967.

78. Yee RD, Foos RY, Straatsma BR: Coagulative necrosis in a malignant melanoma of the choroid at the macula with extensive subretinal hemorrhage. Invest Ophthalmol 12:525-531, 1973.

79. Zakka KA, Foos RY, Spencer WH, et al.: Cavitation in intraocular malignant melanoma. Arch Ophthalmol 100:112-114, 1982.

80. Zimmerman LE: Malignant melanoma of the uveal tract. In Spencer WH (Ed): Ophthalmic Pathology. An Atlas and Textbook, Third Ed. Philadelphia, WB Saunders, 1986, pp 2072-2139.

CHAPTER 5

NATURAL HISTORY

Understanding the natural history of a disease is important not only to make treatment decisions but also to appraise treatment results. Unfortunately, data is limited concerning important natural history issues of choroidal malignant melanoma.[1,15,27,28,30] Traditionally, treatment is done once a diagnosis of malignant melanoma is made. However, because of the uncertainty of the diagnosis of smaller melanocytic lesions, observation for growth is recommended usually. Therefore, there is more natural history information regarding smaller lesions. A small lesion can be defined as less than 10 mm in largest diameter and 2.5 mm in height.

Of eyes with a small melanocytic choroidal lesion, 12% to 55% will show growth when followed from several months to 20 years (**Figs. 5.1, 5.2**).[5,7,8,12–14,24–26] In a series of 116 patients followed prospectively for six to eight years after detection of a suspicious melanocytic lesion, approximately 60% of the tumors (64 small, 4 medium) demonstrated no evidence of growth, whereas 40% (36 small, 7 medium and 5 large) grew.[7,8,12] There were no tumor-related deaths in the group without demonstrable growth (minimum follow-up of 6 years). Seven of the 48 (15%) patients with observed tumor growth died of metastatic disease; three of the seven had large tumors when first seen. This mortality figure is similar to other series in which enucleation was done primarily without definite observation for growth, albeit, comparison between series is difficult. In another series, 20 patients with small melanocytic lesions were followed from two to 20 years.[5] Growth was observed in 11 (55%). In still another series, 37 of 42 (88%) patients with small lesions (measured 3 mm to 7.5 mm in diameter and less than 2 mm in elevation) were observed; all remained unchanged during a minimum period of four years.[21] Medium-sized lesions (defined in this series as larger than $10 \times 10 \times 3$ mm and less than $15 \times 15 \times 5$ mm or 1,125 mm^3) are more likely to grow than small lesions, and growth occurred in about two-thirds of cases in one series.[12]

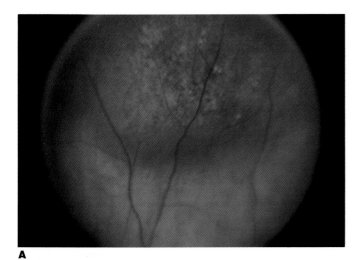

A

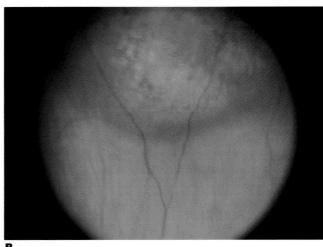

B

Figure 5.1 A & B Large Suspicious Choroidal Nevus
This 61 year-old female was found to have a suspicious choroidal nevus that measured 8 mm in diameter and 1.4 mm thick (Figure 5.1A). No change in size was documented over an 8 year period (Figure 5.1B). Note that the tumor edge is in the same location as indicated by the retinal vessels.

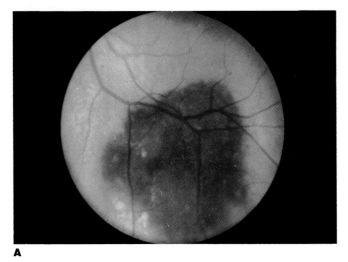
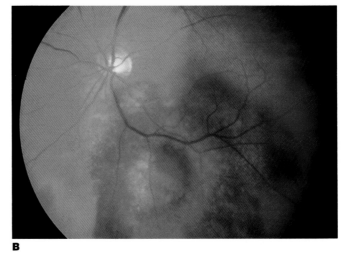

A

B

Figure 5.2 A & B Enlargement Of A Choroidal Pigmented Lesion
This 66 year-old female had a 5 mm suspicious choroidal nevus (Figure 5.2A). Thirteen years later there was definite enlargement (Figure 5.2B).

Various methods can estimate the rate at which malignant melanoma grows. One method, an inferred natural history analysis, assumes that differences in the average age among patients with different stages of a disease represent a time scale of the disease process itself. Such an analysis of 2,105 cases in the Registry of Ophthalmic Pathology determined that, on average, small tumors require approximately two years to grow to a medium size, and five years for a medium-sized tumor to become large.[20] However, information concerning whether or not the tumors had grown prior to enucleation was not available. Many small tumors do not grow for many years.[5,13,26] Moreover, in another series, about one-third of medium-sized lesions (4 of 11) did not grow while observed for a minimum of eight years.[12,13]

Another method for estimation of growth rates calculates tumor volume at two different times.[2,3,12,19] The change in tumor volume with time provides an estimate of the length of time necessary for the tumor to double in volume (tumor doubling time). A faster tumor doubling time for mixed-cell tumors than for spindle-cell tumors has been calculated.[3,12] Another analysis determined that the rate of increase in tumor height was similar for spindle- and for mixed-cell tumors.[4] In contrast, others have concluded that the growth rate for spindle-cell tumors was slightly faster than for mixed-cell tumors.[20]

A division of pigmented ciliochoroidal lesions into two groups has been suggested: Group 1 would represent a characteristic nevus with little or no growth potential; Group 2 would represent a malignant melanoma with both slow-growth and rapid-growth phases.[2] Over variable lengths of time, a malignant melanoma may enter a rapid-growth phase. According to this hypothesis, and though exceptions exist, tumors seen in the slow-growth phase are generally small spindle-cell tumors with a better prognosis, whereas tumors in the rapid-growth phase have a poorer prognosis and are generally medium-sized or larger with a mixed- or epithelioid-cell type. Because epithelioid and mixed-cell tumors are usually larger tumors, the transformation from the slow-growth phase to the rapid-growth phase may be associated with a transformation to a more malignant cell type in the tumor, although small tumors may be mixed or epithelioid cell-type.[9–11,20] The determination of a possible slower growth rate for spindle-cell tumors compared with mixed- and epithelioid-cell tumors supports this hypothesis.[3] Also, faster growth rates for larger tumors have been demonstrated.[12] Additionally, cell culture studies demonstrate the ability of human malignant melanoma cells to transform from spindle-cell type to epithelioid-cell type and back again.[16,23] Another study indicated that cell division is faster, and mitotic index higher, when the cells are epithelioid in appearance.[16] Although unproved, this may offer further support to the concept that epithelioid cells exhibit a faster growth rate. Yet, serial observations of tumors indicate that periods of tumor growth may be interspersed with somewhat dormant intervals.[4,12]

Although the data is very limited on observed growth of small lesions, there is even less information about more advanced, untreated melanomas. An evaluation of a series of 29 patients who had refused treatment, or who had metastatic disease diagnosed at the time of treatment concluded that a malignant melanoma grows slowly over many years before acquiring metastatic potential.[29] But, the detection of metastatic disease is hampered by the limited sensitivity and specificity of currently available tests; one can not assume that metastatic disease is absent because it is not detected. Moreover, the natural history of early metastatic disease is unknown. Can micrometastatic foci remain somewhat dormant for a period of time before growing large enough to produce symptoms and be detected? Is it possible for small metastatic foci to regress completely? The development of more sensitive detection methods of metastatic lesions may provide a better understanding of these questions.

Some have considered that tumor necrosis, possibly induced by an immunological response, may produce tumor regression.[22] Documentation of spontaneous regression is extremely limited.[1,17,18,22] One well-documented case of a presumed malignant melanoma showed growth initially but then apparently complete regression ensued (determined ophthalmoscopically) associated with extensive chorioretinal scarring.[18] Interestingly, a recurrence developed along the edge of the chorioretinal scarring. Subsequent histologic examination showed uveal inflammatory cell infiltration in the area of chorioretinal scarring. Other reported cases have shown regression over variable periods of time (up to 8 years)[6] and with variable degrees of associated uveal inflammatory responses.[17,22]

SUMMARY

The natural history of many small melanocytic lesions suggests little if any growth for several years. Nevertheless, some will grow, and therefore regular observation of these lesions is essential. Those lesions that grow, appear to do so relatively slowly. Once growth is observed, treatment is indicated in most cases.

REFERENCES

1. Albert DM: Ocular melanoma: A challenge to visual science. Friedenwald Lecture. Invest Ophthalmol Vis Sci 23:550-580, 1982.

2. Apple DJ, Blodi FC: Uveal melancytic tumors: A grouping according to phases of growth and prognosis with comments on current theories of nonenucleation treatment. Int Ophthalmol Clin 20:33-61, 1980.

3. Augsburger JJ, Gonder JR, Amsel J, et al.: Growth rates and doubling times of posterior uveal melanomas. Ophthalmology 91:1709-1715, 1984.

4. Char DH, Heilbron DC, Juster RP, Stone RD: Choroidal melanoma growth patterns. Br J Ophthalmol 67:575-578, 1983.

5. Char DH, Hogan MJ: Management of small elevated pigmented choroidal lesions. Br J Ophthalmol 61:54-58, 1977.

6. Chong CA, Gregor RJ, Augsburger JJ, Montana J: Spontaneous regression of choroidal melanoma over 8 years. Retina 9:136-138, 1989.

7. Curtin VT: Choroidal and ciliary body malignant melanomas. Mod Probl Ophthalmol 20:115-120, 1979.

8. Curtin VT, Cavender JC: Natural course of selected malignant melanomas of the choroid and ciliary body. Mod Probl Ophthalmol 12:523-527, 1974.

9. Davidorf FH, Lang JR: The natural history of malignant melanoma of the choroid: small vs. large tumors. Trans Acad Ophthalmol Oto 79:310-320, 1975.

10. Davidorf FH, Lang JR: Small malignant melanomas of the choroid. Am J Ophthalmol 78:788-793, 1974.

11. Flocks M, Gerende JH, Zimmerman LE: The size and shape of malignant melanomas of the choroid and ciliary body in relation to prognosis and histologic characteristics: a statistical study of 210 tumors. Trans Am Acad Ophthalmol Oto 59:740-758, 1955.

12. Gass JDM: Comparison of uveal melanoma growth rates with mitotic index and mortality. Arch Ophthalmol 103:924-931, 1985.

13. Gass JDM: Observation of suspected choroidal and ciliary body melanomas for evidence of growth prior to enucleation. Ophthalmology 87:523-528, 1980.

14. Gonder JR, Augsburger JJ, McCarthy EF, Shields JA: Visual loss associated with choroidal nevi. Ophthalmology 89:961-965, 1982.

15. Graham GJ, Duane TD: Ocular melanoma task force report. Am J Ophthalmol 90:728-733, 1980.

16. Irvine AR, Mannagh J, Arya DV: Change in cell type of human choroidal malignant melanoma in tissue culture. Am J Ophthalmol 80:417-424, 1975.

17. Jensen OA, Anderson SR: Spontaneous regression of a malignant melanoma of the choroid. Acta Ophthalmol 52:173-182, 1974.

18. Lambert SR, Char DH, Howes E, et al.: Spontaneous regression of a uveal melanoma. Arch Ophthalmol 104:732-734, 1986.

19. Manschot WA, van Peperzeel HA: Choroidal melanoma. Enucleation or observation? A new approach. Arch Ophthalmol 98:71-77, 1980.

20. McLean IW, Foster WD, Zimmerman LE, Martin DG: Inferred natural history of uveal melanoma. Invest Ophthalmol Vis Sci 19:760-770, 1980.

21. Mims JL, Shields JA: Follow-up studies of suspicious choroidal nevi. Tr Am Acad Ophthalmol Oto 85:929-943, 1978.

22. Reese AB, Archila EA, Jones IS, Cooper WC: Necrosis of malignant melanomas of the choroid. Am J Ophthalmol 99:104, 1970.

23. Reese AB, Ehrlich G: The culture of uveal melanomas. The Proctor Medal Lecture. Am J Ophthalmol 46:163-174, 1958.

24. Shields JA: Diagnosis and Management of Intraocular Tumors. St. Louis, CV Mosby, 1983.

25. Shields JA, Augsburger JJ: The management of choroidal melanomas. Editorial. Am J Ophthalmol 90:266-268, 1980.

26. Thomas JV, Green WR, Maumenee AE: Small choroidal melanomas. A long-term follow-up study. Arch Ophthalmol 97:861-864, 1979.

27. Zimmerman LE: Metastatic disease from uveal melanomas. A review of current concepts with comments concerning future research and prevention. Tr Ophthalmol Soc UK 100:34-54, 1980.

28. Zimmerman LE, McLean IW: Changing concepts of the prognosis and management of small malignant melanomas of the choroid. Montgomery Lecture, 1975. Tr Ophthalmol Soc UK 95:487-494, 1975.

29. Zimmerman LE, McLean IW: Metastatic disease from untreated uveal melanomas. Am J Ophthalmol 88:524-534, 1979.

30. Zimmerman LE, McLean IW, Foster WD: Statistical analysis of follow-up data concerning uveal melanomas, and the influence of enucleation. Ophthalmology 87:557-564, 1980.

CHAPTER 6

METASTATIC EVALUATION

A careful evaluation for metastatic disease must be performed before a malignant choroidal melanoma is treated (**Table 6.1**).[1,3,38] Compared with patients who have nonocular malignancies, very few patients with malignant posterior uveal melanoma (2.5% in some series) have discernable evidence of metastatic disease when they are first seen.[3,7,20,26,35] A higher incidence figure of 6.5% was reported but this series was later reappraised and additional patients managed over a longer time were included.[41] The reappraisal showed a 2.5% incidence of metastatic disease at the time of diagnosis, which is similar to other studies.[26] Because it is difficult to detect very small metastases, it is likely that some patients have undetected metastatic disease at the time of diagnosis.[8,10,24] It is important to recognize that about 5% to 10% of patients with malignant choroidal melanoma will have a history of nonocular malignancy.[2,16,20]

The most common site of metastatic disease is the liver, which is frequently the only metastatic focus.[4,9,14,18,20,29,34,38,39] Other involved sites include the skin, bone, pleura, brain, lung, pericardium, gastrointestinal tract, lymph nodes, and pancreas.[3,7,14,20,34] Lesions in these sites are rarely found at the time of diagnosis of choroidal melanoma. Detection of most metastases is during the first four to five years following treatment, and approximately half of these are within three years of treatment.[5,18,20–23,30,32,37] Metastases can be diagnosed as long as 42 years following enucleation.[33]

All patients should have a careful, complete physical examination. Patients with metastases may note right upper quadrant pain, fullness, nausea, vomiting, dyspepsia, bone pain, and weight loss.[8,20] Laboratory studies should be tailored with the knowledge that the liver is the most frequent site of metastatic disease, but opinions differ concerning the most appropriate studies.

Good serum screening studies include lactate dehydrogenase (LDH), alkaline phosphatase (AP), gamma-glutamyl transpeptidase (GTP), and aspartate aminotransferase (AST). LDH is very sensitive, and a normal serum LDH level is good evidence of no liver involvement. In one series of 426 patients with metastatic ocular and nonocular malignant melanoma, the LDH false-negative rate was about 2%, and a false-positive result occurred in about 50% of cases.[13] GTP also appears to be a very

sensitive indicator of metastatic disease.[8,10,15,26] In one study, an elevated GTP was predictive of future metastatic disease; when elevated, subsequent metastatic disease occurred in 70% of patients with at least 2 years follow-up,[15] but 30% of patients with an abnormal GTP level were not subsequently found to have metastatic disease. This may change with longer follow-up of these patients. Data from this work has provided evidence that as many as 13% of patients may have metastatic disease at the time of initial diagnosis.[15]

Some recommend routine use of either liver-spleen scans or abdominal CT scans for the metastatic evaluation of patients,[3,26] while others reserve this more comprehensive evaluation for those patients with abnormal liver function studies.[7–9,19,25,38] Despite normal serum liver function studies, some patients may

Table 6.1
Evaluation for Metastatic Disease

Physical examination	Chest x-ray
Subcutaneous nodules	Complete blood count
Cutaneous melanocytic lesions	Serum liver function studies
Liver enlargement	gamma-glutamyl transpeptidase
Lymph nodes	lactate dehydrogenase
Breast	alkaline phosphatase
G.I.	aspartate aminotransferase

Other evaluations as suggested by review of systems

ADDITIONAL EVALUATIONS IF RESULT IS ABNORMAL

Liver abnormality	Breast
abdominal CT scan	mammography
GI	Skin/lymph node
GI series	biopsy
endoscopy	Lung
	CT scan

have metastatic disease that is detectable with a liver-spleen scan or abdominal CT scan.[3,9,12,26] Most clinicians prefer an abdominal CT scan since a liver-spleen scan cannot detect a nodule less than approximately 2.5 cm in size.[8,26] Further evaluations of an abnormality on a liver-spleen scan or abdominal CT scan depend on the clinical situation. Other recommended routine studies include a chest x-ray and complete blood count.[8,26,38]

The unusual and well-documented predilection of malignant melanoma to metastasize to the liver is an interesting phenomenon. A possible explanation for the correlation between an increased serum GTP level and the development of metastatic disease may be a predilection of tumor cells to seed the liver in the presence of pre-existing liver disease.[40] In support of this hypothesis is an experimental study that showed a higher frequency of metastatic disease when liver damage was present.[27] Other experimental work has shown the ability to select a clone of tumor cells with a particular predilection for developing liver metastasis. This suggests selective interactions between binding protein receptors on hepatocytes and tumor cells.[11]

The life expectancy of patients with metastatic choroidal melanoma is short.[7,14,18] The median interval from development of metastasis to death is from three months to eight months,[14,18,20,28] the mean varies from 18 weeks up to 1.3 years,[4,7] and the range is from 3 months to 7 years.[4,7] Life expectancy is significantly shorter with primarily hepatic involvement compared with pulmonary or subcutaneous metastatic lesions.[28] Median survival is better in patients under age 50 to 55 compared with those over age 50 to 55.[18,28]

Treatment of metastatic melanoma is, for the most part, discouraging.[36,38] A recent report, however, described encouraging results for hepatic metastases using embolization of the hepatic artery with polyvinyl sponge and cisplatin.[6] Another approach, although with limited applicability, has been resection of a solitary hepatic metastasis.[17] Adjuvant chemotherapy for patients without metastatic disease undergoing enucleation can be done; a nonrandomized study suggests longer than expected disease-free survival.[31] Further work is necessary to confirm this.

SUMMARY

Prior to treatment of a malignant melanoma, a careful systemic evaluation should be undertaken to survey for possible metastatic disease. Because metastatic disease at the time of diagnosis is infrequently detected, it is likely that microscopic foci are present that are undetectable with currently available studies. Important advances will include more sensitive and specific tests for metastatic disease. Also, since treatment of metastatic disease is in most cases unsuccessful, improved therapeutic options are necessary. This, together with improved and earlier detection of metastatic disease, may allow selection of patients for early systemic treatment to achieve enhanced survival rates.

REFERENCES

1. Abramson DH, Ellsworth RM: Treatment of choroidal melanomas. Bull NY Acad Med 54:849-854, 1978.

2. Albert DM: Ocular melanoma: A challenge to visual science. Friedenwald Lecture. Invest Ophthalmol Vis Sci 23:550-580, 1982.

3. Albert DM, Wagoner MD, Smith ME: Are metastatic evaluations indicated before enucleation of ocular melanoma? Editorial. Am J Ophthalmol 90:429-432, 1980.

4. Birdsell JM, Gunther BK, Boyd TA, et al.: Ocular melanoma: A population-based study. Can J Ophthalmol 15:9-12, 1980.

5. Callender GR, Wilder HC, Ash JE: Five hundred melanomas of the choroid and ciliary body followed five years or longer. Am J Ophthalmol 25:962-967, 1942.

6. Carrasco CH, Wallace S, Charnsangavej C, et al.: Treatment of hepatic metastases in ocular melanoma. Embolization of the hepatic artery with polyvinyl sponge and cisplatin. JAMA 255:3152-3154, 1986.

7. Char DH: Metastatic choroidal melanoma. Am J 7.Ophthalmol 86:76-80, 1978.

8. DH: Clinical Ocular Oncology. New York, Churchill Livingstone, 1989, pp 91-149.

9. Donoso LA, Berd D, Augsburger JJ, et al.: Metastatic uveal melanoma. Pretherapy serum liver enzyme and liver scan abnormalities. Arch Ophthalmol 103:796-798, 1985.

10. Donoso LA, Nagy RM, Brockman RJ, et al.: Metastatic uveal melanoma. Hepatic cell-surface enzymes, isoenzymes, and serum sialic acid levels in early metastatic disease. Arch Ophthalmol 101:791-794, 1983.

11. Donoso LA, Nagy RM, McFall RC, et al.: Metastatic choroidal melanoma. Hepatic binding protein reactivity toward a liver-metastasizing clone. Arch Ophthalmol 101:787-790, 1983.

12. Donoso LA, Shields JA, Augsburger JJ et al.: Metastatic uveal melanoma: Diffuse hepatic metastasis in a patient with concurrent normal serum liver enzyme levels and liver scan. Letter to the Editor. Arch Ophthalmol 103:758, 1985.

13. Einhorn LH, Burgess A, Vallejos C, et al.: Prognostic correlations and response to treatment in advanced metastatic malignant melanoma. Cancer Res 34:1995-2004, 1974.

14. Einhorn LH, Burgess MA, Gottlieb JA: Metastatic patterns of choroidal melanoma. Cancer 34:1001-1004, 1974.

15. Felberg NT, Shields JA, Maguire J, et al.: Gamma-glutamyl transpeptidase in the prognosis of patients with uveal malignant melanoma. Am J Ophthalmol 95:467-473, 1983.

16. Fine SL, Collaborative Ocular Melanoma Study Group: Second non-ocular cancers in patients with choroidal melanoma. Ophthalmology (Suppl) 95:128, 1988.

17. Fournier GA, Albert DM, Arrigg CA, et al.: Resection of solitary metastasis. Approach to palliative treatment of hepatic involvement with choroidal melanoma. Arch Ophthalmol 102:80-82, 1984.

18. Gragoudas ES, Egan KM, Seddon JM, et al.: Survival of patients with metastases from uveal melanoma. Ophthalmology 98:383-390, 1991.

19. Gragoudas ES, Seddon JM, Egan K, et al.: Long-term results of proton beam irradiated uveal melanomas. Ophthalmology 94:349-353, 1987.

20. Jensen OA: Malignant melanomas of the uvea in Denmark 1943-1952. A clinical, histopathological, and prognostic study. Acta Ophthalmol (Suppl) 75:1-220, 1963.

21. Kidd MN, Lyness RW, Patterson CC, et al.: Prognostic factors in malignant melanoma of the choroid: A retrospective survey of cases occurring in Northern Ireland between 1965-1980. Trans Ophthalmol Soc UK 105:114-121, 1986.

22. Lommatzsch P, Dietrich B: The effect of orbital irradiation on the survival rate of patients with choroidal melanoma. Ophthalmologica 173:49-52, 1976.

23. MacRae A: Prognosis in malignant melanoma of choroid and ciliary body. Tr Ophthalmol Soc UK 73:3-30, 1953.

24. Manschot WA, van Peperzeel HA: Choroidal melanoma. Enucleation or observation? A new approach. Arch Ophthalmol 98:71-77, 1980.

25. Miller TR, Gomez-Moreiras JJ, Smith ME et al.: The value of liver scintigraphy in choroidal melanoma. Arch Ophthalmol 97:1875-1876, 1979.

26. Pach JM, Robertson DM: Metastasis from untreated uveal melanoma. Arch Ophthalmol 104:1624-1625, 1986.

27. Pascal SG, Saulenas AM, Fournier GA, et al.: An investigation into the association between liver damage and metastatic uveal melanoma. Am J Ophthalmol 100:448-453, 1985.

28. Rajpal S, Moore R, Karakousis CP: Survival in metastatic ocular melanoma. Cancer 52:334-336, 1983.

29. Reese AB: Pigmented tumors. In Tumors of the Eye. Third Ed, New York, Harper & Row, 1976, pp 173-226.

30. Seddon JM, Albert DM, Lavin PT, Robinson N: A prognostic factor study of disease-free interval and survival following enucleation for uveal melanoma. Arch Ophthalmol 101:1894-1899, 1983.

31. Sellami M, Weil M, Dhermy P, et al.: Adjuvant chemotherapy in ocular malignant melanoma. Oncology 43:221-223, 1986.

32. Shammas H, Blodi FC: Prognostic factors in choroidal and ciliary body melanomas. Arch Ophthalmol 95:63-69, 1977.

33. Shields JA, Augsburger JJ, Donoso LA, et al.: Hepatic metastasis and orbital recurrence of uveal melanoma after 42 years. Am J Ophthalmol 100:666-668, 1985.

34. Terry TL, Johns JP: Uveal sarcoma-malignant melanoma. A statistical study of ninety-four cases. Am J Ophthalmol 18:903-913, 1935.

35. Wagoner MD, Albert DM: The incidence of metastases from untreated ciliary body and choroidal melanoma. Arch Ophthalmol 100:939-940, 1982.

36. Westbury G: Chemotherapy in the treatment of malignant melanomas. Tr Ophthalmol Soc UK 97:445-447, 1977.

37. Westerveld-Brandon ER, Zeeman WPC: The prognosis of melanoblastoma of the choroid. Ophthalmologica 134:20-29, 1957.

38. Willson JKV: Systemic evaluation and management of a patient with a choroidal melanoma. In Schachat AP (Ed): Retina. Tumors, St. Louis, CV Mosby, 1989, vol. 1, pp 729-731.

39. Zakka KA, Foos RY, Omphroy CA, Straatsma BR: Malignant melanoma. Analysis of an autopsy population. Ophthalmology 87:549-556, 1980.

40. Zimmerman LE: Gamma-glutamyl transpeptidase in the prognosis of patients with uveal malignant melanoma. Correspondence. Am J Ophthalmol 96:409-410, 1983.

41. Zimmerman LE, McLean IW: Metastatic disease from untreated uveal melanomas. Am J Ophthalmol 88:524-534, 1979.

CHAPTER 7

MANAGEMENT: GENERAL CONSIDERATIONS AND THE ROLE OF OBSERVATION

Many factors influence the management decisions of malignant melanomas. Treatment choice may depend on the patient's age and health, presence of symptoms, size and location of the melanoma, physician philosophy, and patient preference.

In considering therapeutic options, it is convenient to group malignant melanoma into small, medium, and large tumor groups. A common convention classifies a small melanoma as less than 10 mm in basal diameter and 2.5 mm in elevation, a medium melanoma as 10 mm to 16 mm in basal diameter and 2.5 mm to 8 mm in height, and a large melanoma as exceeding these dimensions. Placing a tumor into one of these size categories helps to guide treatment decisions. But many factors can influence the following guidelines.

OBSERVATION OF SMALL LESIONS

The major dilemma in managing small melanocytic lesions is the difficulty of differentiating a large choroidal nevus (also called benign melanoma or nevoma by some authorities) from a small malignant melanoma (**Fig. 7.1,** page 78). The prognosis for survival of patients with a malignant melanoma correlates closely with the size of the tumor and is very good for small lesions. For this reason, some advocate immediate treatment once a small and suspicious choroidal lesion is recognized.[22,25,30] Other clinicians, however, believe that the uncertain growth potential of small suspicious pigmented lesions dictates that they should be observed and not treated. The current controversies surrounding these opposed methods of management, and also the uncertainty of the diagnosis of these small tumors, leads most to reason that observation for growth, particularly in older individuals, is the better approach. Evidence suggests that this approach permits retention of many eyes with a small lesion and carries little or no risk.[1,2,5–8,17,19,21,29,32–34,37,38]

Several fundamental questions are at the center of the controversy concerning the management of small melanocytic lesions. When in the life cycle of a malignant melanoma does metastatic potential develop and metastasis occur? What is the risk of observing a small melanocytic lesion without immediate treatment? What percent of lesions will subsequently show growth? What factors, if any, will help predict future growth? Unfortunately, definitive answers to these questions are not available but important data can guide our current management.

In a large series of 116 patients that were followed prospectively for six to eight years after detection of a suspicious melanocytic lesion, approximately 60% of the tumors (64 small, 4 medium) showed no evidence of growth, whereas 40% (36 small, 7 medium and 5 large) grew.[9,10,15] There were no tumor related deaths in the group without demonstrable growth (minimum follow-up of 6 years). Seven of the 48 (15%) patients with observed growth of their tumors died of metastatic disease, three of which had large tumors when first seen. This mortality figure is similar to other series in which enucleation was done primarily without a period of observation for evidence of tumor growth, albeit, comparison between series is difficult.

No metastatic deaths occurred in one series[15] with tumors smaller than 180 mm^3, and 98 mm^3 in another series[36] (although metastasis was present in one patient with a tumor less than 98 mm^3). Another series of 20 patients with small melanocytic lesions did not have any tumor-related deaths; volumes were not reported, but all tumors had a diameter of less than 10 mm and a height not greater than 2 mm.[8] Therefore, the volume of the tumors in this series could be estimated as less than 200 mm^3. In still another series of 42 patients with lesions measuring 3 mm to 7.5 mm in diameter and less than 2 mm in elevation (maximum volume approximately 110 mm^3) and observed for growth, no metastatic deaths occurred.[27] These reports suggest that observation of small lesions for growth does not appear to influence prognosis in an unfavorable manner.

In a large series, symptoms were present in 50% of the patients that subsequently showed tumor growth, but only 25% of the patients that showed no tumor growth were symptomatic. Symptoms or signs that correlate with a higher likelihood of

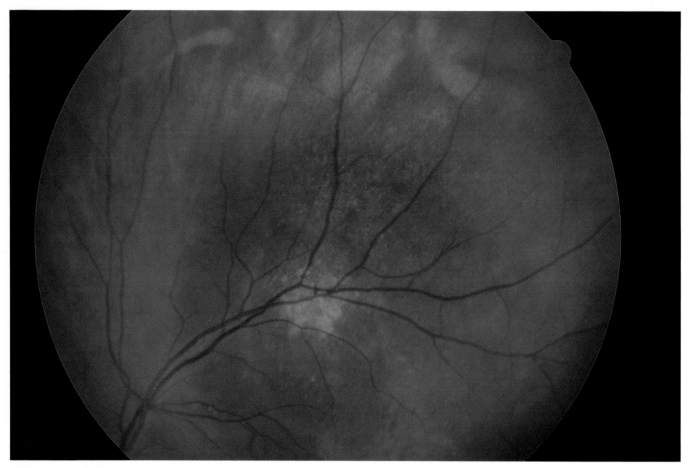

Figure 7.1 Suspicious Choroidal Nevus
This 47 year-old female was found to have an 8 mm × 8 mm diameter pigmented lesion superotemporal to the left optic nerve during a routine examination. Standardized echography measured the maximal height as 1.9 mm. Regular follow-up was recommended. If growth is documented, then treatment is indicated.

future growth include: photopsias;[16] multiple patches of orange pigment **(Fig. 7.2)** over the tumor surface (rather than small patches of orange pigment usually intermingled with drusen);[16,35] intrinsic tumor vessels (more easily seen with fluorescein angiography); and angiographic signs of multiple pinpoint areas of hyperfluorescence **(Fig.7.3,** page 80) that increase in fluorescence during the later phases of the angiogram (in small tumors with little evidence of drusen).[16] A localized serous retinal detachment **(Fig. 7.3)** appears to indicate an increased risk of

growth,[12,16] particularly if the lesion is over 5 mm in diameter and is 2 to 3 mm thick.[12,18,27] Another potential sign of future growth is the presence of a discrete zone of hyperfluorescence over the surface of a melanoma.[23]

Signs that help predict low growth potential of pigmented lesions include multiple drusen **(Fig. 7.4,** page 81) scattered over the surface of the tumor (when examination of the fellow eye reveals absent or insignificant drusen in the corresponding area of the retina) and choroidal neovascularization.[16]

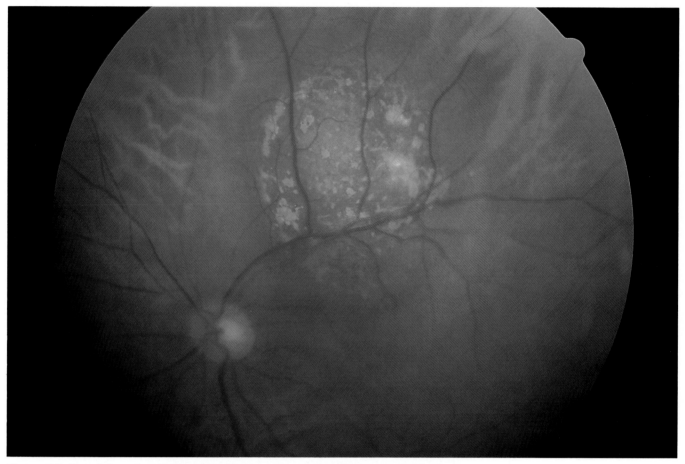

Figure 7.2 Suspicious Small Choroidal Melanocytic Lesion With Orange Pigment
This 71 year-old male had noted blurred vision in this eye for approximately 1 year. The visual acuity was 20/40. Note the multiple patches of orange lipofuscin pigment over the surface that is more suggestive of future growth.

Patients with a small melanocytic lesion should have the size of the lesion carefully documented with a fundus sketch, color photographs, and standardized echography. Fluorescein angiography may provide additional information that can help decide the relative likelihood of future growth. Lesions that are 5 mm or less in largest basal diameter should usually be checked in 4 to 6 months. Larger lesions should be initially checked within 3 to 4 months. Even if no ophthalmoscopic evidence of growth occurs, serial echographic examinations are necessary to document the thickness and to exclude evidence of extraocular extension.

MANAGEMENT OF MEDIUM AND LARGE LESIONS

Treatment options for medium-sized lesions mostly include enucleation, some form of irradiation, and resection (mostly small or small-medium tumors). In general, enucleation is the best treatment for large melanomas. There may be a role for treatment of eyes that contain a large melanoma with low-dose external beam radiation prior to enucleation. Although plaque radiotherapy can treat some large melanomas that are on the smaller side of the large tumor group, and charged particle irradiation

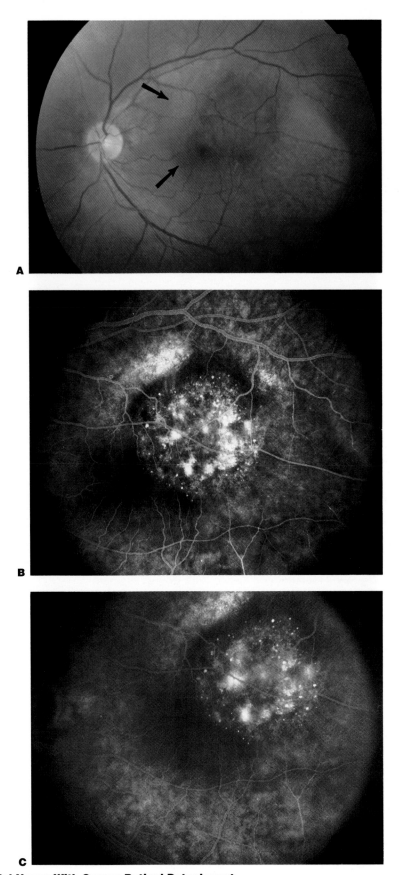

Figure 7.3 A–C Choroidal Nevus With Serous Retinal Detachment
This 60 year-old male was noted to have a pigmented choroidal lesion with an overlying serous retinal detachment (arrows). The visual acuity was 20/32. The fluorescein angiogram (Figs. 7.3B & C) demonstrated multiple pinpoint fluorescein leakage areas.

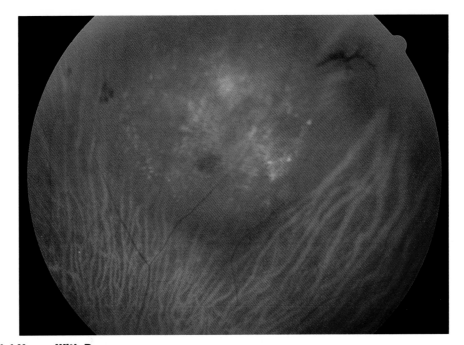

Figure 7.4 Choroidal Nevus With Drusen
This 64 year-old male was noted to have an 8 mm diameter choroidal nevus in his right eye. Note the multiple drusen. Drusen were not present in the corresponding area of the left eye.

can effectively treat even larger melanomas, the chance of salvaging useful vision becomes much less, and the chance of significant radiation complications becomes much higher. Thus, enucleation is recommended frequently for large melanomas.

Because several treatment options for a malignant melanoma may be possible, it is important to inform a patient about the relative efficacy of each treatment option. The goal of ophthalmologists is to preserve vision whenever possible. However, we must shift our perspective to an oncologist's and first consider treatment options in terms of survival.

Recommendations about the best treatment of malignant melanoma vary widely.[2-4,11,13,14,20,26,28,31] Some authorities strongly believe that any management other than enucleation is untenable.[11,24,25] Others consider alternative therapies as equally efficacious in preserving life.[3,31]

Several retrospective studies have attempted to compare different therapies. However, these studies do not conclusively answer the question of which therapy is best because of their retrospective nature and consequent potential for unintentional biases. For this reason, work is currently in progress to study this issue in a prospective, randomized fashion. In England, a national study is underway in which patients with tumors greater than 8 mm in elevation will be randomized to receive either proton beam therapy or enucleation. In the United States, the ongoing Collaborative Ocular Melanoma Study (COMS) is evaluating survival following enucleation or ^{125}I plaque radiotherapy for medium-sized lesions and survival following enucleation alone or supplemented with pre-enucleation external beam radiotherapy for large lesions. Such efforts will provide us with important information with which to counsel our patients.

SUMMARY

The managment of malignant melanomas can be guided by determination of the size of a lesion. For small lesions, since some doubt exists as to whether or not it is truly a malignant melanoma, observation for some evidence of growth is most frequently recommended. Tumors that are medium or large are most frequently treated with some form of radiation therapy or enucleation. Definitive data are not available to determine which form of treatment is optimal of survival.

REFERENCES

1. Abramson DH, Ellsworth RM: Treatment of choroidal melanomas. Bull NY Acad Med 54:849-854, 1978.

2. Albert D: Toward resolving the ocular melanoma controversy. Arch Ophthalmol 97:451-452, 1979.

3. Augsburger JJ: Does treatment improve or worsen the survival rate of patients? Ophthalmology (Suppl) 95:147, 1988.

4. Boniuk M: A crisis in the management of patients with choroidal melanoma. Editorial. Am J Ophthalmol 87:840-841, 1979.

5. Char DH: The management of small choroidal melanomas. Surv Ophthalmol 22:377-386, 1978.

6. Char DH: Clinical Ocular Oncology. New York, Churchill Livingstone, 1989, pp 91-149.

7. Char DH: Therapeutic options in uveal melanoma. Editorial. Am J Ophthalmol 98:796-799, 1984.

8. Char DH, Hogan MJ: Management of small elevated pigmented choroidal lesions. Br J Ophthalmol 61:54-58, 1977.

9. Curtin VT: Choroidal and ciliary body malignant melanomas. Mod Probl Ophthalmol 20:115-120, 1979.

10. Curtin VT, Cavender JC: Natural course of selected malignant melanomas of the choroid and ciliary body. Mod Probl Ophthalmol 12:523-527, 1974.

11. Davidorf FH, McAdoo JF: Enucleation for choroidal melanoma. In: Schachat AP (Ed): Retina. Tumors. Vol. 1. St. Louis, CV Mosby, 1989, pp 687-691.

12. Erie JC, Robertson DM: Serous detachments of the macula associated with presumed small choroidal melanomas. Am J Ophthalmol 102:176-178, 1986.

13. Fine SL: Do I take the eye out or leave it in? Arch Ophthalmol 104:653-654, 1986.

14. Fine SL: Controversy in the management of choroidal and ciliary body melanoma. Ophthalmology (Suppl) 95:147, 1988.

15. Gass JDM: Comparison of uveal melanoma growth rates with mitotic index and mortality. Arch Ophthalmol 103:924-931, 1985.

16. Gass JDM: Observation of suspected choroidal and ciliary body melanomas for evidence of growth prior to enucleation. Ophthalmology 87:523-528, 1980.

17. Gass JDM: Problems in the differential diagnosis of choroidal nevi and malignant melanomas. Am J Ophthalmol 83:299-323, 1977.

18. Gonder JR, Augsburger JJ, McCarthy EF, Shields JA: Visual loss associated with choroidal nevi. Ophthalmology 89:961-965, 1982.

19. Hagler WS, Jarrett WH, Killian JH: The use of the ^{32}P test in the management of malignant melanoma of the choroid: A five-year follow-up study. Tr Amer Acad Ophthalmol Oto 83:49-60, 1977.

20. Jakobiec FA: A moratorium on enucleation for choroidal melanoma? Editorial. Am J Ophthalmol 87:842-846, 1979.

21. Jensen OA: Malignant melanomas of the uvea in Denmark 1943-1952. A clinical, histopathological, and prognostic study. Acta Ophthalmol (Suppl) 75:1-220, 1963.

22. Kersten RC: Management of choroidal malignant melanoma at Iowa. Ophthalmologica 189:24-35, 1984.

23. Leff SR, Augsburger JJ, Shields JA: Focal fluorescence of choroidal melanoma. Br J Ophthalmol 70:104-106, 1986.

24. Manschot WA, Van Strik R: Is irradiation a justifiable treatment of choroidal melanoma? Analysis of published results. Br J Ophthalmol 71:348-352, 1987.

25. Manschot WA, van Peperzeel HA: Choroidal melanoma. Enucleation or observation? A new approach. Arch Ophthalmol 98:71-77, 1980.

26. Maumenee AE: An evaluation of enucleation in the management of uveal melanomas. Editorial. Am J Ophthalmol 87:846-847, 1979.

27. Mims JL, Shields JA: Follow-up studies of suspicious choroidal nevi. Tr Am Acad Ophthalmol Oto 85:929-943, 1978.

28. Packer S: The management of choroidal melanoma. Arch Ophthalmol 102:1450-1451, 1984.

29. Raivio I: Uveal melanoma in Finland. An epidemiological, clinical, histological and prognostic study. Acta Ophthalmol 133:5-64, 1977.

30. Ruiz RS: Early treatment in malignant melanomas of the choroid. In Brockhurst RJ, Boruchoff SA, Hutchinson BT, Lessel S (Eds): Controversy in Ophthalmology. Philadelphia, WB Saunders, 1977, pp 604-610.

31. Shields JA: Counseling the patient with a posterior uveal melanoma. Am J Ophthalmol 106:88-91, 1988.

32. Shields JA: Changing trends in the management of choroidal melanomas. Tr Pac Coast Oto-Ophthalmol So 60:215-225, 1979.

33. Shields JA: Diagnosis and Management of Intraocular Tumors. St. Louis, CV Mosby Co, 1983.

34. Shields JA, Augsburger JJ: The management of choroidal melanomas. Editorial. Am J Ophthalmol 90:266-268, 1980.

35. Smith LT, Irvine AR: Diagnostic significance of orange pigment accumulation over choroidal tumors. Am J Ophthalmol 76:212-216, 1973.

36. Thomas JV, Green WR, Maumenee AE: Small choroidal melanomas. A long-term follow-up study. Arch Ophthalmol 97:861-864, 1979.

37. Zimmerman LE, McLean IW: Changing concepts of the prognosis and management of small malignant melanomas of the choroid. Montgomery Lecture, 1975. Tr Ophthalmol Soc UK 95:487-494, 1975.

38. Zimmerman LE, McLean IW, Foster WD: Does enucleation of the eye containing a malignant melanoma prevent or accelerate the dissemination of tumor cells? Br J Ophthalmol 62:420-425, 1978.

CHAPTER 8

ENUCLEATION

For many years, clinicians believed that the best treatment for malignant melanoma is enucleation. Currently, however, significant controversy exists about its role.[9,34,47] What the role of enucleation is in the management of malignant melanoma, and the determination of the best treatment for malignant melanoma, will require carefully controlled prospective data. Yet, reviewing the available literature provides a foundation for building our understanding of the many complexities of malignant melanoma.

Evidence indicates that several ophthalmoscopic and histologic characteristics (such as largest tumor diameter, tumor location, and histologic cell type) provide important prognostic information. But some tumor characteristics are probably interrelated and therefore may not represent statistically significant independent determinants of prognosis. Multivariate statistical techniques help decide which are independent prognostic factors. Some published reports have used a multivariate analysis and these are discussed in this chapter.

GENERAL PROGNOSIS

The reported five-year survival rate following enucleation ranges from 50% to 75%, and the ten-year survival ranges from 35% to 65% (**Tables 8.1 & 8.2**).[7,12,30,35,40,42,43,48,59,60,65,69,81] Different statistical methods have been used in these reports that makes accurate comparisons difficult. Also, the actual number of patients dying of metastatic disease from malignant melanoma is difficult to know since autopsy or biopsy confirmation is not always done.[29]

PROGNOSIS AND CELL TYPE

The Callender histopathologic tumor classification provides significant prognostic information concerning survival. In many series, the tumor cell type represents the most important factor

(**Table 8.1**, page 84).[7,21,28,30,35,36,40,42,43,48,50,58–61,65,69,79,80,82] Spindle cell tumors have the best prognosis and epithelioid cell tumors have the worst. Mixed-cell tumors are intermediate. Most series classify tumors by specific cell types. Alternatively, the number of epithelioid cells per high-power field (HPF) can be used in lieu of a Callender-type classification. This approach avoids some potential variability of the Callender classification, but pathologists may have different criteria for classifying a cell as epithelioid.

In two reports from the same center, a multivariate analysis determined that the number of epithelioid cells per HPF was the most important prognostic factor for survival.[65,80] However, a multivariate analysis by other researchers showed that cell type was a less important determinant of prognosis than tumor size (see below).[40]

To increase objectivity in classifying tumors, a computerized system of measurement of nucleolar area was developed.[25,27] A larger inverse standard deviation of the nucleolar area (ISDNA) correlates with a better survival. A still better method of predicting survival results when the ISDNA determination is combined with the measurement of the largest tumor diameter (LTD).[26] Both the number of epithelioid cells per HPF and the ISDNA measurement can accurately predict death from metastatic melanoma but the ISDNA is slightly more predictive.[66] Among those patients that eventually die of metastatic disease, the ISDNA may be a better predictor of length of survival than other factors such as the LTD.[19] Finally the ISDNA of tumor cells obtained by fine needle aspiration biopsy can be measured, but does not, unfortunately, appear to provide prognostic information; this is probably due to limited sampling of the tumor.[22]

PROGNOSIS AND TUMOR SIZE

Many studies showing a definite and important relationship between tumor size and mortality have been done (**Table 8.2,** page 85).[21,23,36,40,43,48,58,65,69] Estimates and measurements of the size of a tumor have involved comparisons to the crystalline lens, estimates of the volume by a product of the two basal dimensions

Table 8.1
Prognosis Following Enucleation Related to Histologic Classification

Series	Number	Survival Overall*	Spindle A	Spindle B	Mixed	Epithelioid
Callender et al.[12] F/U: > 5 yrs	500	52%	Combined Spindle A & B: 78%	----	38%	29%
Wilder et al.[82] F/U: > 5 yrs	2,535	55%	89% 81%	77% 64%	37% 22%	33% 0%
Paul et al.[59] F/U: > 5 yrs	2,652	71%	95% 85%	89% 80%	60% 46%	43% 34%
Jensen, 1970[36] F/U: > 15 yrs	230	53%	Combined Spindle A & B: 68%	----	38%	19%
Hagler et al.[31] F/U: > 5 yrs	90	86%	100%	92%	81%	55%
Raivio[60] F/U: > 10 yrs	354	65% 52%	Combined Spindle A & B: 69%	----	66%	53%
Davidorf et al.[16] F/U: > 5 yrs	50	94%	Combined Spindle A & B: 96%	----	75%	100%
Shammas et al.[69] F/U: > 6 yrs	293	N/A†	94%	69%	57%	36%
McLean et al.[48] F/U: > 5 yrs	217	75%	92%	84%	40%	0% Only 2 cases
Barr et al.[5] F/U: > 6 yrs	18	89%	Combined Spindle A & B: 92%	----	Combined Mixed & Epithelioid:	80%
Thomas et al.[78] F/U: median 7.2 yrs	65	95%	Combined Spindle A & B: 95% 15 yr	----	Combined Mixed & Epithelioid	90% (5 year) 80% (10 year)
Packard[58] F/U: > 5 yrs	484	79%	Combined Spindle A & B: 85%	----	58%	57%
Kidd et al.[40] F/U: > 5 yrs	87	72% 56%	Combined Spindle A & B: 76%	----	Combined Mixed & Epithelioid	53%

* 5 year survival unless otherwise indicated; second number is 10 year survival if available.

† N/A: Not available

and the height, or by the product of the largest basal diameter and the height, and also other methods.[21,30,43]

In 1955, Flocks and associates reported the first attempt at a quantitative determination of a relationship between tumor size (tumor volume) and mortality.[21] Tumor volume (determined by the product of three dimensions) over 1344 mm^3 had a poorer prognosis (46% alive five or more years after enucleation) than those eyes with a tumor volume less than 1344 mm^3 (88% alive five or more years after enucleation). Surprisingly, they could not show a relationship between prognosis and volume when considering those tumors with a volume less than 1344 mm^3. Note that in this study small tumors were classified as less than 1344 mm^3, whereas today a tumor of this size is considered a large tumor.

More frequently today, the largest tumor diameter is used and provides important prognostic information for survival.[36,40,48,58,65,69]

A multivariate analysis of a series of patients showed that tumor volume was an important independent prognostic factor (the largest tumor diameter had a similar significance).[40] Clearly, some measure of tumor bulk provides important prognostic information.

Diffuse melanomas have a particularly poor survival prognosis; the five-year survival was 27% in one series.[23] These are also more frequently associated with extraocular extension.

Tumor Size, Cell Type and Prognosis

Larger tumors are more frequently classified as epithelioid, mixed-cell, or necrotic,[5,21,28,40] though not all series agree.[37] Large spindle A or B, or fascicular tumors, have a better prognosis than large epithelioid, mixed-cell, or necrotic tumors.[21,28,48,58] For instance, tumors with a largest tumor diameter over 10 mm and a mixed- or epithelioid-cell type were shown to have a 36% survival compared with 82% for spindle-cell tumors of this size.[48] Likewise, mixed- or epithelioid-cell type tumors with a largest tumor diameter less than 10 mm had a 53% survival compared with 93% for spindle cell tumors. Additionally, larger tumors within a given cell classification had a poorer prognosis; for example, larger spindle A, B, or fascicular tumors had a poorer prognosis than smaller spindle A, B, or fascicular tumors.[21]

Tumor height correlates with prognosis to a certain extent as well. A taller tumor has a worse prognosis for survival, but this is correlated with a larger tumor diameter.[69] Those tumors with less than 3 mm of elevation have a better prognosis than tumors over 3 mm in height.[48] Yet, others conclude that tumor elevation is not an independent predictor of outcome.[65]

PROGNOSIS AND TUMOR LOCATION

Tumors with an anterior border located anterior to the equator have a poorer prognosis than more posterior tumors.[28,48,58,60,65,69] Peripapillary tumors have a somewhat poorer prognosis as well,

Table 8.2
Prognosis Following Enucleation Related to Tumor Size

Series	Number	Overall Survival[*]	< 10 mm[†]	> 10 mm
Callender et al.[12] F/U: > 5 yrs	500	52%	N/A[‡]	N/A
Wilder et al.[82] F/U: > 5 yrs	2,535	55%	N/A	N/A
Westerveld-Brandon[81] F/U: > 5 yrs	103	69%	N/A	N/A
Paul et al.[59] F/U: > 5 yrs	2,652	71%	N/A	N/A
Jensen, 1970[36] F/U: > 15 yrs	230	53%	58% < 100 mm² basal area	N/A
Font et al.[23] F/U: < 1 up to > 10 yrs	54	27%	- - - -	All diffuse tumors
Hagler et al.[31] F/U: > 5 yrs	90	86%	95%	83%
Raivio[60] F/U: > 10 yrs	354	65% 52%	Basal Areas:	< 38 mm²: 67% 38 to 74 mm²: 77%
Davidorf et al.[16] F/U: > 5 yrs	50	94%	94%	None in series
Shammas et al.[69] F/U: > 6 yrs	293	N/A	87%	30% (LTD > 12 mm)
McLean et al.[48] F/U: > 5 yrs	217	75% 64%	80%	61%
Barr et al.[5] F/U: > 6 yrs	18	89%	89%	None in series
Thomas et al.[78] F/U: median 7.2 yrs	65	95%	95%	None in series
Seddon et al.[65] F/U: 8 up to 28 yrs	267	74% 63%	89%	35% (LTD > 15 mm)
Packard[58] F/U: > 5 yrs	484	79%	N/A	N/A
Kidd et al.[40]	87	72% 56%	N/A	50% (Tumor vol: > 900 mm³)

[*] 5 year survival, except where indicated otherwise; second number indicates 10 year survival if available.
[†] Largest tumor diameter.
[‡] N/A: Not available.

though the difference is small and not statistically significant.[80] Confounding both observations is the more frequent finding of larger tumors in an anterior or peripapillary location.[30,65,69,80] Still, although more anterior tumors tend to have a largest tumor diameter greater than 10 mm, both tumor location and the largest tumor diameter appear to be independent predictors of survival.[66]

PROGNOSIS, EXTRAOCULAR EXTENSION AND EXENTERATION

Extraocular tumor extension occurs in 7% to 28% of cases (note that extension outside the globe is differentiated from some degree of intrascleral extension). Prognosis for survival is worse when malignant melanoma extends outside the globe **(Fig. 8.1)** and the orbital recurrence rate is higher (10% to 23%).[1,6,16–18,30,31,35,40,48,56,58,60,61,71,76,79] In one series, the five-year survival of patients with extraocular extension was 27% compared with a five-year survival rate of 78% in those patients without extraocular extension.[71] Careful inspection of the globe at the time of enucleation is essential to ensure that an area of extraocular extension is not transsected.[10] Most commonly, extraocular tumor extension occurs with larger or diffuse melanomas,[23,61,71,86] though rarely, patients with somewhat small tumors have had prominent extraocular masses.[14,20,71,86] Also, extraocular extension has occurred in eyes with a small melanoma under observation and that clinically showed little or no intraocular change in tumor size.[64] Extrascleral extension is more frequently associated with epithelioid, mixed-cell, or necrotic tumors.[42,71,76,80,86] The diameter or volume of the extraocular tumor has correlated with survival in some reports[40,56,76] but not all.[1,71]

Optic Nerve Invasion

Peripapillary tumors more frequently invade the optic nerve or subarachnoid space.[61,70] Prelaminar or retrolaminar optic nerve invasion occurs in 54% to 62% of reported peripapillary tumors **(Fig. 8.2)**, and subarachnoid invasion in about 16% to 46% of cases.[70,80] If, however, we consider choroidal and ciliary body melanomas in all locations within the eye, and not just those

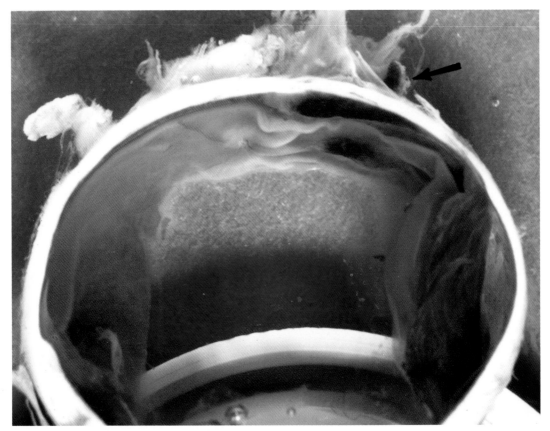

Figure 8.1 Malignant Melanoma And Extrascleral Extension
This 79 year-old female was noted to have a growing melanoma and extraocular extension was suspected by ultrasonography (Figure 2.4) and CT scan (Figure 2.12). This was confirmed at the time of enucleation. Note the pigmented tumor outside the globe (arrow).

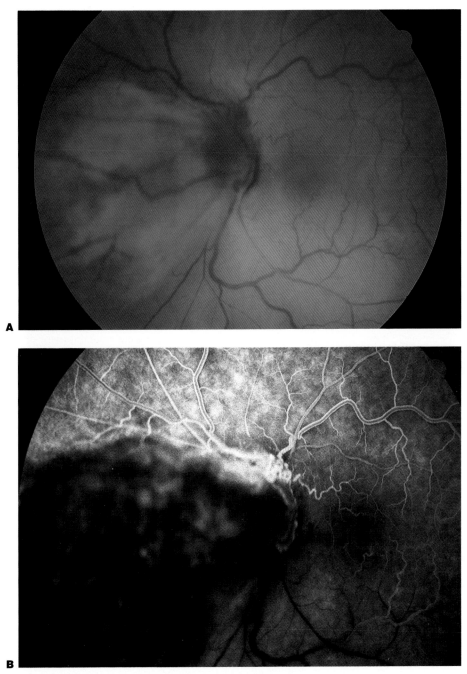

Figure 8.2 A & B Malignant Melanoma Causing Retinal Artery Occlusion

This 66 year-old man noted reduced vision in his left eye. He had an 8 mm × 11 mm peripapillary melanoma that measured 4.6 mm in thickness. The fluorescein angiogram (Figure 8.2B) shows occlusion of the inferior branches of the central retinal artery. Despite the apparent invasion of the optic nerve, histologic examination showed that this melanoma extended only to the level of the lamina cribosa. Serial sections showed that tumor compression of the retinal arteries produced the artery occlusion rather than tumor invasion of the arterial wall.

with peripapillary involvement, optic nerve or subarachnoid invasion occurs in only 1% to 14% of cases.[1,35,48,61,70,80]

Optic nerve invasion is more likely in an eye with absent light perception, glaucoma, tumor necrosis, and retinal invasion.[70,75] Rarely, optic nerve invasion can follow posterior seeding of ciliary body or iris tumor.[75] Optic nerve and subarachnoid invasion is more commonly associated with epithelioid or mixed-cell tumors.[70,80]

Invasion of the optic nerve beyond the lamina cribrosa has a worst prognosis: a 67% to 83% mortality rate when present compared with a 30% to 50% mortality rate when absent.[1,35,48,80] But disagreement exists about prelaminar optic nerve extension representing a significantly worse prognostic sign.[1,48]

Orbital Recurrence

Orbital tumor recurrence is more common in eyes with extraocular tumor extension and most patients with an orbital tumor recurrence succumb to metastatic disease.[1,71,76] The role of exenteration for the management of extraocular extension is controversial.[1,14,35,71–73,76] Although exenteration is not likely to be curative, even if done within two months of enucleation,[39,71] some argue that there may be a slightly better survival for nonencapsulated or transsected extensions, but most believe that exenteration does not produce a survival benefit.[1,35,56] Exenteration probably should be considered as a palliative procedure.[76]

The excision of a localized orbital nodule and surrounding tissues (tenonectomy) is a useful and practical alternative to exenteration.[14,56,72–74,83,84] In cases of limited extrascleral extension, preenucleation radiation therapy should be considered[73,74] or alternatively, orbital radiotherapy can follow enucleation.[33] In the rare occurrence of massive orbital extension, delay of palliative exenteration until absolutely necessary is suggested; adjunct preoperative or postoperative radiation therapy (50 Gy to 60 Gy) may be considered.[63]

PROGNOSIS AND MITOTIC FIGURES

The number of mitotic figures per HPF correlates with prognosis, tumor doubling time (time required for a tumor to double in volume), and a growing tumor before enucleation.[5,28,48,65] Some work suggests that the prognosis for survival is worse when two or more mitotic figures per 40 HPF are present,[48] but others conclude that the number of mitotic figures relates to the number of epithelioid cells per HPF and is not an independent risk factor.[65] Still, the relationship between the number of mitotic figures and histologic classification is not clear. More mitotic figures within a tumor have correlated with the presence of more epithelioid cells in some reports[4,65] but not other series.[5,28] Finally, melanomas that are observed to grow prior to enucleation appear to have more mitotic figures per HPF than melanomas that do not grow before enucleation.[5]

ADDITIONAL PROGNOSTIC FACTORS

Various factors have been investigated and have variable degrees of significance for prognosis. These include DNA content abnormalities in tumors, patient age, the presence of Bruch's membrane rupture, tumor pigmentation, and the extent of reticulin fibers within the tumor.

An abnormal number of chromosomes (aneuploidy) within tumor cells, that is, DNA content abnormalities, correlates with survival for reasons that are not fully understood. In a series of 79 patients with at least five years of follow-up, survival was worse when DNA content abnormalities were more severe.[52]

The exact relationship of patient age with prognosis is not clear but it appears that patients over age 60 have a poorer prognosis than younger patients.[40,58–60,65,81] Yet, not all evaluations have concluded this, noting better survival only in females under age 40,[36] or a worse survival for patients over age 60 only if the largest tumor diameter is greater than 10 mm.[58] In those eyes with extraocular tumor extension, an earlier onset of metastatic death may correlate with an older age.[1]

Although some reports conclude that the presence of a Bruch's membrane rupture correlates with a worse prognosis,[60,69] others have not shown this.[21,35] Despite these reports, rupture of Bruch's membrane probably does not suggest a worse prognosis but relates to the size of the tumor that in turn correlates with survival.[58] That is, as a tumor enlarges, it is more likely to develop a Bruch's membrane rupture than will a smaller tumor.

Although Callender and Wilder noted that heavier tumor pigmentation suggested a poorer survival rate, they concluded that their results were not definitive.[12] A worse prognosis associated with heavy tumor pigmentation has been confirmed in some series,[7,36,43,58,60,65] was prognostic for only spindle cell tumors,[48] or was not prognostic at all in other series.[40] In all of these reports, the degree of pigmentation has been determined histologically and not ophthalmoscopically.

Callender and Wilder also noted a better prognosis for survival when a melanoma contained an extensive network of reticulin fibers compared with those tumors with fewer reticulin fibers.[11] The five-year survival rate for patients with tumors with a heavy reticulin fiber content was 90% compared with 20% for patients with tumors with no reticulin fibers; grades between were associated with an intermediate prognosis.[12] Others have not shown an improved prognosis associated with more reticulin fibers.[36,43,58,60] Indeed, the Armed Forces Institute of Pathology no longer evaluates the extent of reticulin fibers within melanomas.[86]

PROGNOSIS AND MULTIVARIATE ANALYSIS

As this discussion shows, many factors considered individually appear to have prognostic significance but frequently are interrelated. Therefore, a multivariate analysis of risk factors is necessary to determine which factors are most important for predicting prognosis. One multivariate analysis found that when four factors are considered, the best predictors, in order of significance, are cell type, largest tumor diameter, scleral extension, and the presence of two or more mitotic figures per 40 HPF.[48] A second report found that the five most important prognostic factors in order of importance are: the number of epithelioid cells per HPF, the largest tumor diameter, the location of the anterior tumor border, optic nerve involvement at the line of transection, and the degree of pigmentation.[65]

ENUCLEATION AND POSSIBLE TUMOR CELL DISSEMINATION

The possible benefit of enucleation has been debated since the late 1800s.[3] In 1978, Zimmerman, McLean, and Foster raised concerns that enucleation of an eye with a malignant melanoma may promote and accelerate tumor cell dissemination,[90] a concept that had been experimentally investigated earlier.[24] This concern originated because of the observation that metastatic disease at the time of diagnosis of a malignant melanoma is unusual, about 2%, whereas, the mortality increases abruptly two to three years following enucleation, to about 8%. Also, observing patients with a malignant melanoma for a period of time before removing the eye (because of the physician's philosophy or because of patient refusal for enucleation) is rarely associated with the development of metastatic disease prior to treatment.[57,87,89] Thus, the provocative concept that enucleation may be harmful rather than beneficial was put forth.[85,87,90,91] Nonetheless, this speculation has met with significant counterarguments, suggesting other explanations for the apparent increase in mortality after enucleation.[2,9,15,28,34,38,44-46,49,51,62,67,68,88]

Evaluation of the mortality curve following enucleation for malignant melanoma shows similarity, for the most part, to the shape of mortality curves associated with many nonocular tumors following either radiation or surgical therapies.[67] Some argue that patients in reported series were diagnosed or treated because of the onset of symptoms that represented an accelerated growth phase. Also, some argue that analyzing tumor doubling times and growth rates can explain the increase in post-enucleation mortality without hypothesizing surgically-induced tumor cell dissemination.[9,28,34,38,44,46] Furthermore, some authors observe that the growth rates of ocular malignant melanomas are too slow to produce death within two years if metastasis occurs at the time of enucleation.

A few experimental studies lend some support to the Zimmerman and colleagues hypothesis. With a hamster model of an intraocular tumor, a shortened survival is associated with a traumatic enucleation compared with an atraumatic enucleation.[24] Moreover, dramatic increases in intraocular pressure occur during various maneuvers performed during an enucleation; an observation that has led to the development of various techniques to minimize the pressure variations or to freeze the tumor before enucleation (the so-called "no-touch enucleation").[8,24,32,41,53,77] In a comparison of the prognosis of patients treated with a "gentle enucleation" at one hospital with the prognosis of patients treated with enucleation at other hospitals (the exact surgical details were not known), metastatic deaths appeared to occur earlier in those patients treated elsewhere but the overall survival was not statistically significantly different.[54] Immunologic studies of an experimental mouse eye tumor model demonstrates that enucleation combined with suppression of cell-mediated immunity produces a higher rate of metastasis whereas enucleation alone did not appear to increase metastasis.[55]

Lengthy and multiple discussions about enucleation for malignant melanoma have been exchanged. Perhaps we can conclude, as did Siegel and associates, by quoting Robert Frost:

"We dance round in a ring and suppose,
but the Secret sits in the middle and knows."[68]

REFERENCES

1. Affeldt JC, Minckler DS, Azen SP, Yeh L: Prognosis in uveal melanoma with extrascleral extension. Arch Ophthalmol 98:1975-1979, 1980.

2. Albert D: Toward resolving the ocular melanoma controversy. Arch Ophthalmol 97:451-452, 1979.

3. Albert DM: Ocular melanoma: A challenge to visual science. Friedenwald Lecture. Invest Ophthalmol Vis Sci 23:550-580, 1982.

4. Augsburger JJ, Gonder JR, Amsel J, et al.: Growth rates and doubling times of posterior uveal melanomas. Ophthalmology 91:1709-1715, 1984.

5. Barr CC, Sipperley JO, Nicholson DH: Small melanomas of the choroid. Arch Ophthalmol 96:1580-1582, 1978.

6. Barry DR: Malignant melanoma of the choroid. A review of the histopathology of 100 cases. Trans Ophthalmol Soc UK 93:647-664, 1973.

7. Benjamin B, Cumings JN, Goldsmith AJB, Sorsby A: Prognosis in uveal melanomas. Br J Ophthalmol 32:729-747, 1948.

8. Blair CJ, Guerry RK, Stratford TP: Normal intraocular pressure during enucleation for choroidal melanoma. Arch Ophthalmol 101:1900-1902, 1983.

9. Boniuk M: A crisis in the management of patients with choroidal melanoma. Editorial. Am J Ophthalmol 87:840-841, 1979.

10. Brownstein S, Aedy L: Extraocular extension of malignant melanoma of the uvea. Can J Ophthalmol 18:45-48, 1983.

11. Callender GR, Wilder HC: Melanoma of the choroid: The prognostic significance of argyrophil fibers. Am J Cancer 2:251-258, 1935.

12. Callender GR, Wilder HC, Ash JE: Five hundred melanomas of the choroid and ciliary body followed five years or longer. Am J Ophthalmol 25:962-967, 1942.

13. Canny CLB, Shields JA, Kay ML: Clinically stationary choroidal melanoma with extraocular extension. Arch Ophthalmol 96:436-439, 1978.

14. Char DH: Clinical Ocular Oncology. New York, Churchill Livingstone, 1989, pp 91-149.

15. Davidorf FH: Treatment of malignant melanoma. Letter to the Editor. Arch Ophthalmol 97:975-976, 1979.

16. Davidorf FH, Lang JR: The natural history of malignant melanoma of the choroid: Small vs. large tumors. Trans Acad Ophthalmol Oto 79:310-320, 1975.

17. Davies WS: Malignant melanomas of the choroid and ciliary body. A clinicopathologic study. Am J Ophthalmol 55:541-546, 1963.

18. Donders PC: Malignant melanoma of the choroid. Trans Ophthalmol Soc UK 93:745-751, 1973.

19. Donoso LA, Augsburger JJ, Shields JA, et al.: Metastatic uveal melanoma. Correlation between survival time and cytomorphometry of primary tumors. Arch Ophthalmol 104:76-78, 1986.

20. Duffin RM, Straatsma BR, Foos RY, Kerman BM: Small malignant melanoma of the choroid with extraocular extension. Arch Ophthalmol 99:1827-1830, 1981.

21. Flocks M, Gerende JH, Zimmerman LE: The size and shape of malignant melanomas of the choroid and ciliary body in relation to prognosis and histologic characteristics: A statistical study of 210 tumors. Trans Am Acad Ophthalmol Oto 59:740-758, 1955.

22. Folberg R, Augsburger JJ, Gamel JW, et al.: Fine-needle aspirates of uveal melanomas and prognosis. Am J Ophthalmol 100:654-657, 1985.

23. Font RL, Spaulding AG, Zimmerman LE: Diffuse malignant melanoma of the uveal tract: A clinicopathologic report of 54 cases. Tr Amer Acad Ophthalmol Oto 72:877-894, 1968.

24. Fraunfelder FT, Boozman FW, Wilson RS, Thomas AH: No-touch technique for intraocular malignant melanomas. Arch Ophthalmol 95:1616-1620, 1977.

25. Gamel JW, McLean IW: Modern developments in histopathologic assessment of uveal melanomas. Ophthalmology 91:679-684, 1984.

26. Gamel JW, Greenberg RA, McLean IW, et al.: A clinically useful method for combining gross and microscopic measurements to select high-risk patients after enucleation for ciliochoroidal melanoma. Cancer 57:1341-1344, 1986.

27. Gamel JW, McLean I, Grenberg RA et al.: Objective assessment of the malignant potential of intraocular melanomas with standard microslides stained with hematoxylin-eosin. Hum Pathol 16:689-692, 1985.

28. Gass JDM: Comparison of uveal melanoma growth rates with mitotic index and mortality. Arch Ophthalmol 103:924-931, 1985.

29. Gass JDM: Problems in the differential diagnosis of choroidal nevi and malignant melanomas. Am J Ophthalmol 83:299-323, 1977.

30. Greer H, Buckley C, Buckley J, et al.: An Australian choroidal melanoma survey. Factors affecting survival following enucleation. Aust J Ophthalmol 9:255-261, 1981.

31. Hagler WS, Jarrett WH, Killian JH: The use of the ^{32}P test in the management of malignant melanoma of the choroid: A five-year follow-up study. Tr Amer Acad Ophthalmol Oto 83:49-60, 1977.

32. Hidayat AA, LaPiana FG, Kramer K, et al.: The effect of rapid freezing on uveal melanomas. Am J Ophthalmol 103:66-80, 1987.

33. Hykin PG, McCartney ACE, Plowman PN, Hungerford JL: Postenucleation orbital radiotherapy for the treatment of malignant melanoma of the choroid with extrascleral extension. Br J Ophthalmol 74:36-39, 1990.

34. Jakobiec FA: A moratorium on enucleation for choroidal melanoma? Editorial. Am J Ophthalmol 87:842-846, 1979.

35. Jensen OA: Malignant melanomas of the uvea in Denmark 1943-1952. A clinical, histopathological, and prognostic study. Acta Ophthalmol (Suppl) 75:1-220, 1963.

36. Jensen OA: Malignant melanomas of the human uvea. Recent follow-up of cases in Denmark, 1943-1952. Acta Ophthalmol 48:1113-1128, 1970.

37. Kakebeeke-Kemme HM, Oosterhuis JA, de Wolff-Rouendaal D: Five-year follow-up study of choroidal and ciliary body melanomas after enucleation. In Oosterhuis JA (Ed): Ophthalmic Tumors. Dordrecht, Junk Publishers, 1985, pp 9-26.

38. Kersten R, Blodi F: Letter to the editor. Ophthalmology 92:303-306, 1985.

39. Kersten RC, Tse DT, Anderson RL, Blodi FC: The role of orbital exenteration in choroidal melanoma with extrascleral extension. Ophthalmology 92:436-443, 1985.

40. Kidd MN, Lyness RW, Patterson CC, et al.: Prognostic factors in malignant melanoma of the choroid: A retrospective survey of cases occurring in Northern Ireland between 1965-1980. Trans Ophthalmol Soc UK 105:114-121, 1986.

41. Kramer KK, La Piana FG, Whitmore PV: Enucleation with stabilization of intraocular pressure in the treatment of uveal melanomas. Ophthalmol Surg 11:39-43, 1980.

42. Lommatzsch P, Dietrich B: Survival rate of patients with choroidal melanoma. Ophthalmologica 173:453-462, 1976.

43. MacRae A: Prognosis in malignant melanoma of choroid and ciliary body. Tr Ophthalmol Soc UK 73:3-30, 1953.

44. Manschot WA: The natural history of uveal melanomas and its therapeutic consequences. Doc Ophthalmol 50:83-89, 1980.

45. Manschot WA, van Peperzeel HA: Reply to letter to editor. Arch Ophthalmol 98:1301-1303, 1980.

46. Manschot WA, van Peperzeel HA: Choroidal melanoma. Enucleation or observation? A new approach. Arch Ophthalmol 98:71-77, 1980.

47. Maumenee AE: An evaluation of enucleation in the management of uveal melanomas. Editorial. Am J Ophthalmol 87:846-847, 1979.

48. McLean IW, Foster WD, Zimmerman LE: Prognostic factors in small malignant melanomas of the choroid and ciliary body. Arch Ophthalmol 95:48-58, 1977.

49. McLean IW, Foster WD, Zimmerman LE: Choroidal melanoma. Letter to the editor. Arch Ophthalmol 98:1298-1301, 1980.

50. McLean IW, Foster WD, Zimmerman LE: Uveal melanoma: Location, size, cell type, and enucleation as risk factors in metastasis. Hum Pathol 13:123-132, 1982.

51. McLean IW, Zimmerman LE, Foster WD: Letter to the editor. Am J Ophthalmol 88:794-796, 1979.

52. Meecham WJ, Char DH: DNA content abnormalities and prognosis in uveal melanoma. Arch Ophthalmol 104:1626-1629, 1986.

53. Migdal C: Choroidal melanoma: The role of conservative therapy. Tr Ophthalmol Soc UK 103:54-58, 1983.

54. Migdal C: Effect of the method of enucleation on the prognosis of choroidal melanoma. Br J Ophthalmol 67:385-388, 1983.

55. Niederkorn JY: Enucleation-induced metastasis of intraocular melanomas in mice. Ophthalmology 91:692-700, 1984.

56. Pach JM, Robertson DM, Taney BS, Martin JA et al.: Prognostic factors in choroidal and ciliary body melanomas with extrascleral extension. Am J Ophthalmol 101:325-331, 1986.

57. Packard RBS: In malignant choroidal melanoma will a delay in radical treatment influence prognosis? Tr Ophthalmol Soc UK 103:49-53, 1983.

58. Packard RBS: Pattern of mortality in choroidal malignant melanoma. Br J Ophthalmol 64:565-575, 1980.

59. Paul V, Parnell L, Fraker M: Prognosis of malignant melanomas of the choroid and ciliary body. Int Ophthalmol Clin 2:387-402, 1962.

60. Raivio I: Uveal melanoma in Finland. An epidemiological, clinical, histological and prognostic study. Acta Ophthalmol 133:5-64, 1977.

61. Reese AB: Pigmented tumors. In Tumors of the Eye. Third Ed. New York, Harper & Row, 1976, pp 173-226.

62. Reese LT: Enucleation of uveal melanomas. Letter to the editor. Am J Ophthalmol 88:793, 1979.

63. Rini FJ, Jakobiec FA, Hornblass A, et al.: The treatment of advanced choroidal melanoma with massive orbital extension. Am J Ophthalmol 104:634-640, 1987.

64. Ruiz RS: Early treatment in malignant melanomas of the choroid. In Brockhurst RJ, Boruchoff SA, Hutchinson BT, Lessel S (Eds): Controversy in Ophthalmology. Philadelphia, WB Saunders, 1977, pp 604-610.

65. Seddon JM, Albert DM, Lavin PT, Robinson N: A prognostic factor study of disease-free interval and survival following enucleation for uveal melanoma. Arch Ophthalmol 101:1894-1899, 1983.

66. Seddon JM, Polivogianis L, Hseih CC, et al.: Death from uveal melanoma. Number of epithelioid cells and inverse SD of nucleolar area as prognostic factors. Arch Ophthalmol 105:801-806, 1987.

67. Seigel D, Myers M, Ferris F, Steinhorn SC: Survival rates after enucleation of eyes with malignant melanoma. Am J Ophthalmol 87:761-765, 1979.

68. Seigel D, Myers M, Ferris F, Steinhorn SC: Reply to letter to the editor. Am J Ophthalmol 88:797, 1979.

69. Shammas H, Blodi FC: Prognostic factors in choroidal and ciliary body melanomas. Arch Ophthalmol 95:63-69, 1977.

70. Shammas HF, Blodi FC: Peripapillary choroidal melanomas. Extension along the optic nerve and its sheaths. Arch Ophthalmol 96:440-445, 1978.

71. Shammas HF, Blodi FC: Orbital extension of choroidal and ciliary body melanomas. Arch Ophthalmol 95:2002-2005, 1977.

72. Shields JA: Changing trends in the management of choroidal melanomas. Tr Pac Coast Oto-Ophthalmol So 60:215-225, 1979.

73. Shields JA: Diagnosis and Management of Intraocular Tumors. St. Louis, CV Mosby Co, 1983.

74. Shields JA, Augsburger JJ, Dougherty MJ: Orbital recurrence of choroidal melanoma 20 years after enucleation. Am J Ophthalmol 97:767-770, 1984.

75. Spencer WH: Optic nerve extension of intraocular neoplasms. Am J Ophthalmol 80:465-471, 1975.

76. Starr HJ, Zimmerman LE: Extrascleral extension and orbital recurrence of malignant melanomas of the choroid and ciliary body. Int Ophthalmol Clin 2:369-385, 1962.

77. Sudarsky RD, Jakobiec FA, Rodriguez-Sains R, Poole T: Induced ocular hypertension prior to enucleation for choroidal melanoma. Ophthalmology 88:31A-33A, 1981.

78. Thomas JV, Green WR, Maumenee AE: Small choroidal melanomas. A long-term follow-up study. Arch Ophthalmol 97:861-864, 1979.

79. Warren RM: Prognosis of malignant melanomas of the choroid and ciliary body. In Blodi FC (Ed): Current Concepts in Ophthalmology. Vol. 4. St. Louis, CV Mosby, 1974, pp 158-167.

80. Weinhaus RS, Seddon JM, Albert DM, et al.: Prognostic factor study of survival after enucleation for juxtapapillary melanomas. Arch Ophthalmol 103:1673-1677, 1985.

81. Westerveld-Brandon ER, Zeeman WPC: The prognosis of melanoblastomata of the choroid. Ophthalmologica 134:20-29, 1957.

82. Wilder HC, Paul EV: Malignant melanoma of the choroid and ciliary body: A study of 2,535 cases. Mil Surg 109:370-379, 1951.

83. Wolter JR: Tenonectomy. Treatment of epibulbar extension of choroidal melanomas. Arch Ophthalmol 86:529-533, 1971.

84. Wolter JR: Epibulbar extension of malignant choroidal melanoma treated with tenonectomy. Ophthalmic Surg 5:48-52, 1974.

85. Zimmerman LE: Metastatic disease from uveal melanomas. A review of current concepts with comments concerning future research and prevention. Tr Ophthalmol Soc UK 100:34-54, 1980.

86. Zimmerman LE: Malignant melanoma of the uveal tract. In Spencer WH (Ed): Ophthalmic Pathology. An Atlas and Textbook. Ed. 3. Philadelphia, WB Saunders, 1986, pp 2072-2139.

87. Zimmerman LE, McLean IW: An evaluation of enucleation in the management of uveal melanomas. Am J Ophthalmol 87:741-760, 1979.

88. Zimmerman LE, McLean IW: Reply to letter to the editor. Am J Ophthalmol 88:793-794, 1979.

89. Zimmerman LE, McLean IW: The natural course of untreated uveal melanomas. Doc Ophthalmol 50:75-82, 1980.

90. Zimmerman LE, McLean IW, Foster WD: Does enucleation of the eye containing a malignant melanoma prevent or accelerate the dissemination of tumor cells? Br J Ophthalmol 62:420-425, 1978.

91. Zimmerman LE, McLean IW, Foster WD: The Manschot-van Peperzeel concept of the growth and metastasis of uveal melanomas. Doc Ophthalmol 50:101-121, 1980.

CHAPTER 9

RADIATION THERAPY

The goal of radiation treatment is to destroy or to render a tumor incapable of cell division or metastatic spread. Secondary goals are preservation of the eye and as much vision as possible. Radiation therapy appears to produce tumor regression through several mechanisms.[15,16,25,50,53,59,100,103,121,123] Direct damage to the tumor cell's nuclear DNA is probably the most important effect; damaged DNA prevents further cell division and cell death occurs during subsequent mitosis.[15,16,18,50,59,118] This is called tumor cell sterilization.

A cell's radiosensitivity relates to the cell cycle: highest during mitosis and lowest during the interphase portion of the cell cycle.[15,59,121] Because the intermitotic phase of melanoma cells is relatively long, cell death, which is clinically observed as regression of the tumor, may be delayed for several months.[15,50,53]

Another probable radiation-induced effect is damage or destruction of the tumor's vasculature and blood supply caused by radiation injury to vascular endothelial cells.[15,50,53,118,119] Finally, some theorize that an immune response to the tumor tissue may augment the radiation treatment.[100,103] Yet, the immunology associated with malignant melanoma is complex, and the role of the immune system is not certain.[39,61,89]

Responsiveness of a cell to radiation relates to the degree of tissue hypoxia. Radiosensitivity relates inversely to the oxygenation of the tissue.[53,59,74,121] This is particularly important since more hypoxic cells are present in tumor tissue than in normal tissue. Dividing the radiation dosage into several treatment sessions, called dosage fractionation, not only permits some tumor cells to become more oxygenated between treatments but also allows for normal tissue to repair sublethal damage. External beam radiotherapy uses this strategy.

The Relative Biologic Effectiveness (RBE) of a type of radiation permits comparison of different radiation sources and their effectiveness.[59] The RBE is the radiation dose that is necessary to produce a certain tissue effect compared with a reference source, taken to be 250 kV x-rays. Because the RBE is comparative only in evaluating a given tissue effect, it will vary according to different tissue responses.

Radiation therapy for the management of intraocular tumors dates to the early 1900's. Foster Moore, from his early efforts at St. Bartholomew's Hospital in London, encouraged Stallard, who began extensive work in this area in the 1930's.[81,112] Initially, radon seeds were used for the treatment of selected intraocular neoplasms and were inserted directly into the tumor through the sclera. This technique was abandoned in favor of suturing the seeds to the sclera overlying the tumor.[114] This too was unsatisfactory because it produced uneven radiation. Stallard achieved a more even radiation dose distribution when, in 1948, he began to use radium-loaded (radon is a decay product of radium) plaques made from platinum and molded to the curvature of the sclera. Lugs on the sides allowed the plaque to be sutured to the sclera. Stallard subsequently loaded these plaques with ^{60}Cobalt (^{60}Co).

Despite reports in the literature that described malignant melanomas as radioresistant, treatment of melanomas by Stallard, using these ^{60}Co applicators, produced definite tumor regression and preservation of vision in many patients.[111,113,115] Stallard, in citing his experience, commented that it was indeed unfortunate that choroidal melanomas had been described as radioresistant, a term that suggests they are unsuitable for radiation therapy. Instead, his experience showed that choroidal melanomas were amenable to radiation treatment but required somewhat more radiation to produce an effect than other tumors, such as retinoblastoma.[115]

TREATMENT RESPONSE: EVALUATION AND FEATURES

Clinical evaluation of therapeutic response following radiation therapy is done most commonly with serial examination with indirect ophthalmoscopy, fundus photography, and ultrasound measurement of tumor size. Other methods, such as cell cycling studies of material obtained by fine needle aspiration biopsy, have been undertaken in a few cases.[19,21]

Resorption of subretinal fluid usually occurs within six to nine months and is an early sign of a treatment response.[15,71,75,78,100,119] Initially, in some patients, an exudative reaction may produce an increase in the subretinal fluid and surrounding lipid exudate.[15,34,71] Attenuation and closure of choroidal vessels and retinal vessels overlying the melanoma also may be an early observation.[15,76,78,115] Reduction in tumor height occurs later.

Physicians have varied in their definition of an adequate treatment response. Stallard considered adequate treatment to be complete regression of the treated tumor to a flat pigment-stippled scar, which occurred in most cases. During his early efforts, still, he enucleated two eyes, three and ten months following treatment, because of a persistent "prominent" pigmented mass.[115] Histological examination showed primarily pigmented debris. Stallard concluded that the enucleation of these two eyes was premature: one year or longer may be required for tumor regression following radiation of larger tumors. Others also have defined a successful result as total regression to a completely flat scar.[8,75] But a common current standard is some evidence of tumor regression or absence of continued tumor growth.[34,100] The average melanoma following ^{60}Co plaque radiotherapy shows an approximately 50% reduction in height 54 months after treatment and essentially no change in the basal diameter.[29]

Some eyes following radiation treatment have been enucleated because of radiation-induced complications or continued tumor growth. Histopathologic examination has shown variable degrees of tumor cell viability, tumor necrosis, and number of mitotic figures.[18,20,27,36,47,58,67,77,103,117,123] Interpretation of these findings is difficult, particularly when one considers the histopathology of malignant melanomas in eyes without prior radiation treatment; variability of the extent of tumor necrosis and of the number of mitotic figures is very common. It is not known what the growth and metastatic potential of tumor cells that appear viable histologically. Cell culture and DNA cell-cycle studies of eyes that received helium ion treatment[19] or 2,000 rads of pre-enucleation external beam therapy[19,23,] suggest reduced, though not absent, proliferative potential.

RADIATION SOURCES AND CHARACTERISTICS

Several different types of radiation are used to treat malignant melanoma. These include radioactive seeds ([222]Radon, [60]Cobalt, [125]Iodine, [198]Gold, [106]Ruthenium, [192]Iridium, [182]Tantalum) placed in scleral applicators, and charged particle external beams (proton and helium ion).[33,87,89,96,97,111] Sources of radiation for scleral applicators have different characteristics, such as particle energy, type of emitted particles, and half-life. The characteristics of charged particle radiation are discussed later in this chapter (page 101).

The amount of a radioisotope is specified in terms of activity (decays per second), expressed in millicuries or, more recently, megabecquerels.[33] The dose at a given distance from equal activities (millicuries) of a radioisotope depends on the type of particle emitted (e.g. gamma or beta) and the number and energy of these particles. Tissue penetration relates to the energy of an isotope and the type of particle it emits.

Most commonly, the apical height of a tumor determines the radiation dose. Plaque radiation (brachytherapy) delivers significantly higher radiation doses to tissues closer to the plaque than to those that are more distant. For example, the radiation dose used by Stallard in most of his cases ranged from 7,000 to 14,000 rads to the tumors' apex while the dose to the tumors' base ranged from 18,000 to 36,000 rads.[115] To treat adequately the apex of a taller tumor, the base of the tumor will receive more radiation than the base of a less elevated tumor.

The original ophthalmic experience was with [222]Radon. This high energy isotope (energy range: 0.22 to 2.2 meV) has a short half-life of 3.8 days,[89] which prevents reuse of the plaque for subsequent patients. The most extensive ocular experience is with [60]Cobalt, a high-energy (1.17 to 1.33 meV) gamma particle emitter, though some energy emits as beta particles. The platinum casing of the plaque shields the beta particles. Because of the high energy of the gamma particles, 11 mm of lead reduce the radiation dose by only 50%, a characteristic that prevents shielding of noninvolved surrounding ocular and adnexal tissues.[87,89,96,97] The half-life is 5.2 years, which allows multiple reuses of the applicator.[89,97]

[125]Iodine is a lower energy gamma particle emitter (0.027 to 0.035 meV) with a half-life of 60 days.[87,89,96,97] The relatively short half-life limits reuse of the radioactive seeds. Gold is used for the casing of Iodine plaques. The gold of the iodine plaque casing blocks the lower energy gamma particles emitted by the iodine seeds and can effectively shield structures behind the plaque.[33,87,89,96,97]

[106]Ruthenium is a beta particle emitter with an energy range of 2.0 to 3.54 meV and a half-life of 1.0 year.[71] The tissue penetration of this isotope is less than other isotopes; the radiation dose decreases to about 50% at a 3 mm tissue depth.[71] While this characteristic limits the size of tumors that can be treated, the rapid fall-off of radiation helps to limit the exposure of surrounding ocular tissues.[60,71,118] [106]Ruthenium plaques are constructed with a thicker layer of silver on their posterior edge that effectively shields the tissues behind the plaque.[71] [192]Iridium is a gamma emitter with an energy range of 0.296 meV to 0.612 meV and a half-life of 74 days. Shielding this isotope is not feasible. [198]Gold has been used to a lesser extent.[9,83] It is both a beta and gamma particle emitter with an energy level of 0.411 meV and a half-life of 2.7 days. Platinum, encasing each radioactive seed, shields the beta rays, but the gamma rays are not shielded behind the plaque.

Radiation Plaque Therapy Technique

Placement of a plaque requires localizing the tumor borders on the sclera and suturing the plaque (**Fig. 9.1**) to the sclera so that there is a treatment border of approximately 2 mm.[15,41,86,87,89,96,97] The position of the plaque relative to the tumor margins is verified with indirect ophthalmoscopy and transillumination. Also, intraoperative echography can be used for localization and confirmation (**Fig. 9.2**) of the plaque's position.[15,43,86,88,90,91,98,120] Currently, radiation dosages are approximately 8,000 to 10,000 rads to the tumor apex.[33,71,86,89,100,110,116] Depending on the activity

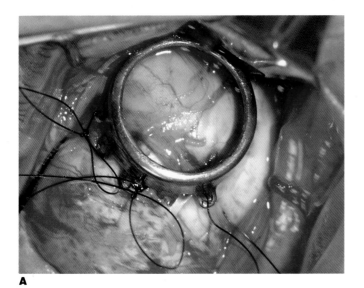

A

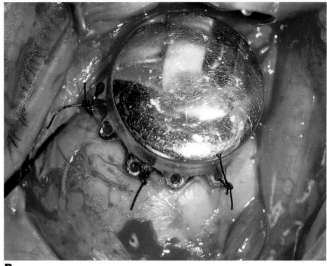

B

Figure 9.1 A & B Placment of Iodine Plaque

A "dummy plaque" that is a metal ring that is the same size and shape as the [125]Iodine loaded plaque has been sutured on the eye. This dummy plaque allows exact placement of sutures and confirmation of the accuracy of placement without exposure to the radiation. This is replaced with the [125]Iodine loaded plaque and secured with the previously placed sutures (Figure 9.1B). This [125]Iodine plaque has a back surface and rim made with gold for radiation shielding purposes.

and type of isotope used, the plaque must be in place approximately four to 14 days to deliver this radiation dose. The plaque is then removed after this period of time.

Cobalt Plaque Radiotherapy

Tables 9.1 and 9.2 summarize the treatment results of most reported series.[8,20,29,34,35,74–76,78,80,100,110,125,127] A brief review of Stallard's results is interesting for historical purposes. In 1968, he published results of the first 107 patients he had treated with radioactive plaques between 1939 and 1964.[115] Successful treatment (considered as regression of the tumor to a flat, pigment-stippled scar) occurred in 78% of patients. Eighteen patients (17%) underwent enucleation because of a poor radiation response. Stallard divided this series of patients into groups, according to the size of the lesion. Treatment success was most frequent in those eyes with a smaller tumor (**Table 9.1**, page 96). Complications are listed in **Table 9.2** (page 97). Stallard concluded that the results were encouraging when the melanoma measured 8 mm or less in diameter and there was no evidence of Bruch's membrane rupture (collar-button formation).

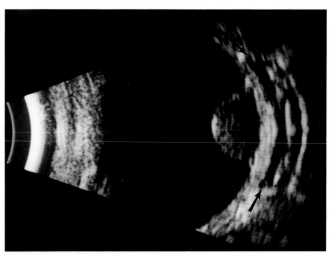

Figure 9.2 Intraoperative Ultrasound Confirmation of Plaque Placement

B-scan ultrasonography can be used intraoperatively to document and confirm the position of the plaque relative to the tumor borders. Note the dark area posterior to the tumor (arrows) that is caused by the plaque (Photo courtesy of Sandra Frazier-Byrne, Miami, FL).

Table 9.1
Cobalt Plaque Results

Report	Number	Size (Diam)	Tumor Regression	Enucleation	5-Year Survival
Stallard[115] F/U: 1 to 25 yrs	107	< 7.5 mm	89%	11%	----
		> 7.5 mm (periphery visible)	77%	20%	----
		7.5 mm (periphery not visible)	64%	18%	----
OVERALL			78%	17%	N/A*
Rotman et al.[100] F/U: min. 3 yrs	24	N/A	N/A	13%	N/A
Char et al.[20] F/U: 3 to 5 yrs	8	6 to 12 mm	67%†	50%	N/A
MacFaul[75] F/U: 2.5 to 17 yrs	107	N/A	65%‡	35%	86%§
Ellsworth[35] F/U: up to 9 yrs	47	3 to 18 mm	N/A	6%	89%
Shields et al.[110] F/U: 1 to 5 yrs	100	5 to 20 mm	96%	2%	79%§
Migdal[80] F/U: min. 5 yrs	99	up to 15 mm	77%‡	23%	95%
Zygulska-Mach et al.[127]	93	up to 15 mm	62%	24%	86%
Zografos et al.[125] F/U: 5 to 13 yrs	60	N.A.	83%	35%	92%¶
Gass[47] F/U: 5 to 16 yrs	21	6 to 19 mm	79%	24%	50%

* N/A: Not available.

† Two patients not included with vitreous hemorrhage following treatment and subsequently enucleated.

‡ More patients may have regressed; figure calculated from number of eyes with complications and lack of tumor control combined.

§ 5-year survival figure taken from another publication from the same group.

¶ Among 60 patients followed for at least 5 years.

It is difficult to appraise accurately the number of eyes that were successfully treated in different series because treatment response following radiation has been judged, managed, and reported differently. For example, enucleation was done in some centers when incomplete tumor regression was observed, whereas others consider arrest of further growth a satisfactory response. Nevertheless, tumor regression has been reported in approximately 65% to 96% of patients.[20,47,75,80,89,100,110]

The rate of tumor regression may be faster in an eye observed to have a more rapidly growing tumor prior to treatment.[7] Additionally, the use of a computerized ultrasound technique suggests that tumors with ultrasonic characteristics that correlate with spindle B tumors may regress more rapidly than mixed-epithelioid cell tumors.[26]

Local tumor recurrence rates are approximately 10% to 12%.[62,124,125] Significant risk factors for the development of a local tumor recurrence include a larger basal diameter and proximity to the optic nerve. Patient survival may be worse when tumor recurrence occurs as compared with patients with good local tumor control, though this probably reflects greater pretreatment risk factors, such as larger tumor size. Difficulty with local control in larger tumors may be a reflection of inadequate radiation treatment along the tumor margin in some of these cases. Also, placing a plaque close to the nerve to treat a peripapillary tumor is difficult since the meningeal coats make the nerve much thicker just posterior to the globe. This may prevent adequate radiation treatment to the edge closest to the nerve. A notched plaque may help this situation. Rarely, tumor recurrence may develop in a noncontiguous location.[32] Recurrences can be treated with enucleation, retreatment with a radioactive plaque, and photocoagulation.[47,75,80,108,110,125] Tumor recurrence can occur as many as nine years following initially successful therapy.[124,125]

The histopathologic findings in 59 patients who underwent enucleation following cobalt plaque therapy was recently

Table 9.2
Cobalt Plaque Complications

Report	F/U	Cataract	Rad. Ret. Optic Neur.	Vit. Heme	Glaucoma	Scleral Necrosis	Keratitis	Misc.
Stallard[115]	1 to 25 yrs	9%	10%	3%	3%	2%	2%	0%
Rotman et al.[100]	at least 3 yrs	N/A*	N/A	N/A	N/A	13%	N/A	N/A
MacFaul[75]	2.5 to 17 yrs	Complications or failure to control tumor led to enucleations in 35% of survivors; complications not listed separately						
Char et al.[20]	3 to 5 yrs	N/A	63%	25%	N/A	N/A	N/A	N/A
Ellsworth[35]	up to 9 yrs	N/A	6%	6%	N/A	2%	N/A	4% (Uveitis)
Shields et al.[110]	1 to 5 yrs	7%	30%	11%	N/A	2%	N/A	7%
Migdal[80]	at least 5 yrs	29%	24%	6%	N/A	N/A	N/A	6%†
Zygulska-Mach et al.[127]	3 to 10 yrs	70%	60%	N/A	35%	N/A	N/A	27%‡
Zografos et al.[125]	5 to 13 yrs	N/A	N/A	12%	2%	N/A	N/A	N/A
Gass[47]	5 to 16 yrs	19%	10%	19%	5%	0%	5%	14%

* N/A: Not available

† Glaucoma, scleral necrosis and miscellaneous grouped together.

‡ Retinal hemorrhages.

reported.[109] The most common reasons for enucleation were tumor recurrence (51%) and neovascular glaucoma (31%). The largest tumor diameter and mitotic activity were significantly greater in the group enucleated because of tumor recurrence than for neovascular glaucoma.

Most available survival data following cobalt-60 radiotherapy has not been adjusted for variable lengths of follow-up. Furthermore, tumors with different risk factors for metastatic death (such as size and location) have been included in different series.[35,75,100,110,115] Life table analysis in some series has determined that the five-year survival rate is between 50% and 75%.[4,47]

Factors related to a poorer prognosis following radiation treatment are similar to those reported following enucleation. These include larger basal diameter, more anterior tumor location, and ciliary body involvement.[4,47,100,110,115] Also, evidence suggests that patients with a tumor that does not decrease in size following treatment have a poorer prognosis.[1] Although one study is frequently interpreted as determing that more rapid tumor regression following treatment is a poor prognostic sign for survival, this work in fact did not show a relationship between percent change in size (height) of a melanoma following treatment and prognosis.[5]

Factors that are predictive of visual loss following radiation treatment include tumor proximity to the fovea and the optic nerve.[115,125] Since radiation complications may take many years to manifest fully, series with shorter follow-up should have better visual acuity results. Occasionally, early visual improvement may occur in some eyes because of resorption of subretinal fluid.

In one series of eyes with an initial visual acuity of 20/25 or better, the cumulative actuarial three-year retention of 20/200 or better visual acuity was 81%; 62% of eyes retained 20/50 or better.[28] Also, eyes subjected to less than 50 Gy (5,000 rads) of radiation to the fovea, the optic nerve, or both, had a significantly better chance of retaining 20/200 or better visual acuity. Medium or large tumors within 5 mm of these structures invariably receive greater than 50 Gy to either, or both, of these structures. Furthermore, large melanomas are at highest risk of developing profound visual loss during the first three years following irradiation treatment. This is most often due to radiation retinopathy involving the fovea. Treatment of a larger tumor (presumably thicker as well) exposes the eye to more radiation; recall that the radiation dose is calculated according to the thickness of the tumor. Lateral spread of the radiation results in increased exposure to the macula and nerve, even when the tumor is more peripheral. In another series, complications did not occur when the macula received a dose of over 200 Gy, whereas severe complications occurred when the optic nerve received this dose.[125]

Other work indicates that approximately 30% to 50% of patients have a visual acuity of 20/60 or better following treatment.[47,75,80,110,115] These figures were lower in some series because

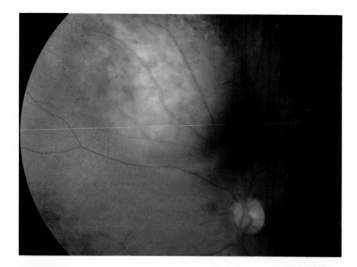

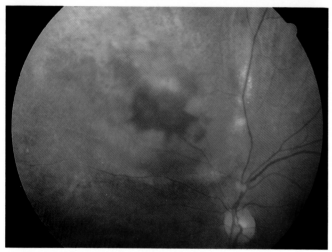

Figure 9.3 A & B Malignant Melanoma Regression Following Radiation Treatment

This 43 year-old female was found to have a superonasal choroidal melanoma (Figure 9.3A). The maximal thickness was 4.4 mm. Two years following ^{125}Iodine plaque irradiation (Figure 9.3B), the thickness had decreased to 2.9 mm and the visual acuity remained 20/20. Note the early signs of radiation retinopathy with cotton wool spots, exudate and hemorrhage.

some eyes were enucleated due to poor tumor control and only surviving eyes were reported.

Complications in these series have varied in reported frequency as well (**Table 9.2**, page 97). These include radiation-induced retinal vasculopathy, optic neuropathy, cataract, vitreous hemorrhage, rubeosis and secondary glaucoma, uveitis, keratitis, punctal occlusion, diplopia, lash loss, and scleral necrosis.[108]

Iodine-125 Plaque Therapy

Features of ^{125}Iodine that make it theoretically a better isotope for ocular brachytherapy include the lower energy of emitted gamma particles. This permits shielding of orbital structures with the gold backing of the plaque. These characteristics have led the Collaborative Ocular Melanoma Study and others to choose this isotope.[33] The use of the isotope, however, has begun somewhat recently and therefore treatment results have less follow-up than available for cobalt.

Tumor regression following ^{125}Iodine plaque therapy occurs in approximately 93% to 96% of cases (**Fig. 9.3**).[46,88] On average, tumors shrink approximately 46% in thickness. This local tumor control rate of over 90% and tumor shrinkage of approximately 50% is similar to results with Cobalt plaques therapy.[29,110]

Early results show a metastatic death rate of up to 17%.[46,88] Complications (**Figs. 9.4, 9.5, 9.6**, pages 99 to 101) include radiation induced retinopathy (17% to 31%), vitreous hemorrhage (14% to 18%), cataract (12% to 25%), glaucoma (10%), and 8% to 14% of eyes were enucleated for tumor growth or complications.[46,85,88] Cataract extraction in selected patients can greatly improve the visual acuity in many patients but in some cases, radiation damage to the macula or optic nerve limits visual improvement.[38]

Preliminary results show that the visual acuity remains within two lines of pretreatment visual acuity in about 55% of patients.[46,88] Visual acuity loss is more common when the tumor margin is within 3-disc diameters of the optic nerve, fovea, or both. In those eyes with a tumor margin within 3 mm of the disc, fovea, or both,[46] the visual acuity remains within two lines of the pretreatment visual acuity in 75% of patients one year following treatment. But by five years following treatment, a steady decline of vision has occurred such that only 43% remain within 2 lines of their pretreatment visual acuity.[85]

Recently, a series of 136 patients, randomized to receive either ^{125}I plaque radiotherapy or helium ion charged particle irradiation (Charged Particle Radiation Treatment, page 101), was reported.[17] In the ^{125}I group, radiation retinopathy was more frequent; external and anterior segment complications were more frequent in the charged particle group. The frequency of metastatic disease in the two treatment groups was similar.

Ruthenium Plaque Therapy

Lommatzsch introduced the use of ^{106}Ruthenium for the treatment of choroidal melanomas in 1964[71]. Because this isotope has limited tissue penetration, tumors that are most suitable for treatment are less than 5 mm to 6 mm thick.[69,71,118] Treatment of larger tumors, however, can be done.[60] Although Lommatzsch uses a radiation dose of approximately 100 Gy (10,000 rads) to the apex, others use different regimens such as 700–800 Gy (70,000 to 80,000 rads) to the tumor base despite the size of the tumor, or 150–200 Gy (15,000 to 20,000 rads) to the tumor apex.[12,13,60,69,71–73,118] Sometimes, radiation treatment is repeated or augmented with photocoagulation.

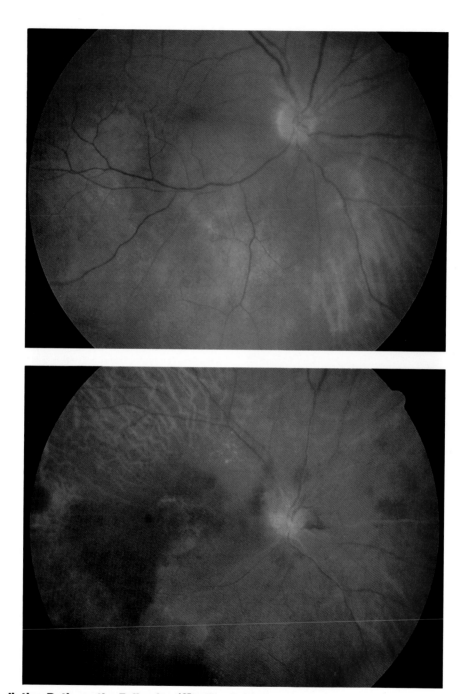

Figure 9.4 A & B Radiation Retinopathy Following ¹²⁵Iodine Radiation Treatment

This 53 year-old female had a choroidal melanoma that measured 5.7 mm thick (Figure 9.4A). She underwent ¹²⁵Iodine plaque irradiation. Approximately 18 months later, the tumor measured 2.2 mm thick and radiation retinopathy was apparent (Figure 9.5B). Note the retinal hemorrhage, cotton-wool spots, retinal exudate and optic nerve swelling. Visual acuity is hand motion.

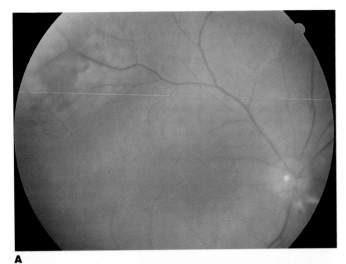

A

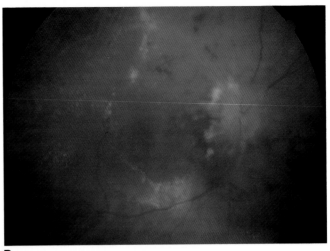

B

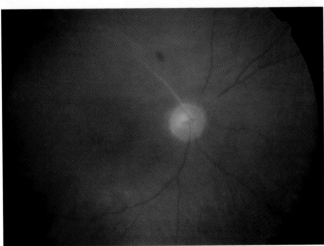

C

Figure 9.5 A–C Radiation Retinopathy Following ¹²⁵Iodine Radiation Treatment

This 57 year-old male presented with a 14 mm diameter choroidal melanoma that measured 6.7 mm thick. Visual acuity was 20/20. ¹²⁵Iodine plaque irradiation treatment was done. One year later (Figure 9.5A), note the peripapillary cotton-wool spots. Two years after radiation treatment, marked progression of the radiation retinopathy was present (Figure 9.5B). Note the retinal hemorrhages, exudate and cotton-wool spots. Thirty-three months after radiation treatment (Figure 9.5C), the hemorrhage and exudate had resolved and the optic nerve had become pale and the retinal vessels appeared sclerotic. The tumor had regressed to a height of 2.4 mm.

Lommatzsch has acquired extensive experience with this isotope and recently described his 20-year experience (**Table 9.3**, page 102).[72,73] Two hundred and twenty-seven patients (followed for at least five years) were reported and of these, 146 (64.3%) were successful (tumor regression with no regrowth and no metastasis).[73] Because this isotope has limited tissue penetration, treatment of smaller tumors with this isotope is most ideal, treatment results of less elevated tumors are most interesting. The melanoma was 5 mm or less in elevation in 175 (77%) of the total of 227 eyes; in these eyes with smaller tumors, treatment produced a flat scar in 97 (55%), partial regression in 38 (22%), no change in approximately 16 (9%), and continued growth in 18 (10%). In the complete series, about 15% of eyes showed continued tumor growth following treatment. Light coagulation was used to enhance the therapeutic response in 24 (10.6%) cases, and 14 cases (6%) had a second radiation plaque treatment. The five- and ten-year survival rate from metastatic death was 88%

and 80%, respectively.[73] Other series have shorter follow-up and therefore slightly more favorable results (**Table 9.3**).

The frequency of enucleation for tumor recurrence or radiation complications is highest in those series with longer follow-up after radiation treatment. Enucleation was necessary in 59 (26%) of 227 patients in Lommatzsch's series (minimum of five years follow-up): 48 because of new tumor growth and 11 because of radiation complications.[73] Other series with shorter follow-up have reported that 3% to 11% of eyes were enucleated.[12,40,60]

Approximately one-third of eyes beginning with 20/40 or better vision have retained this level of visual acuity,[72,118] and approximately 50% of patients retain 20/100 or better.[60] Tumor proximity to the optic nerve or macula requires substantial radiation exposure to these structures. Similar to cobalt and iodine radiation, high doses of ruthenium radiation to the optic nerve or macula is a risk factor for visual loss.

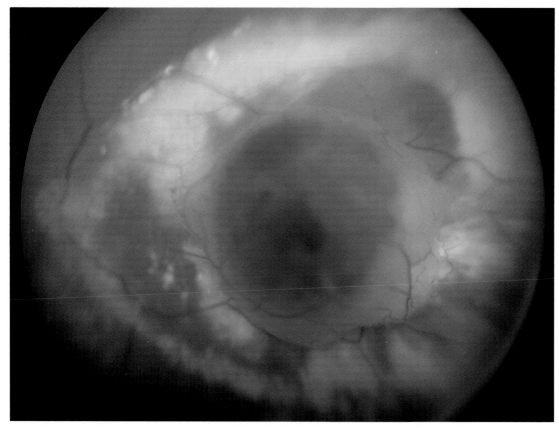

Figure 9.6 Massive Exudate Following ^{125}Iodine Radiation Treatment
This 31 year-old male underwent ^{125}Iodine plaque irradiation approximately 12 months earlier. His pretreatment appearance is shown in Figure 1.9B. Note the deposition of subretinal exudate surrounding the tumor. This leakage appears to have come from the tumor mass.

Complications seen in these series are similar to other reports with different isotopes and include radiation retinopathy and optic neuropathy, scleral necrosis, vitreous hemorrhage, secondary glaucoma, and cataract.[12,40,60,73,118] In one survey of 295 patients followed for up to 5 years, early complications included transitory increase in exudative retinal detachments in 14% of eyes and a radiation-induced anterior uveitis in 4%. Later complications included development of radiation retinopathy (defined as radiation-induced retinal damage away from the tumor area) in 11% of patients; this occurred on average 14.5 months after treatment. Optic neuropathy, glaucoma, vitreous hemorrhage was found in 4%, 2%, and 7%, respectively. No eyes developed rubeosis. An advantage of the limited tissue penetration of the ruthenium isotope is reduced radiation exposure to the lens; cataracts develop in 3% of patients and occurred only in eyes with ciliary body tumors.[40]

Other Isotopes

Other isotopes that have been used include ^{198}gold (^{198}Au, combined with xenon arc photocoagulation) and radon.[9,31,83,84] The experience with radon demonstrated significant radiation com-

plications and visual loss. ^{198}Au treatment achieved tumor control in about 85% of cases with similar visual acuity results as with other isotopes.

Charged Particle Radiation Characteristics and Treatment Technique

External beam therapy with charged particle radiation (proton beam and helium ions) has been used for the treatment of choroidal melanomas.[11,25,57,126] Several advantages have been cited for this form of radiation therapy. Among these are a good control of aiming the beam, minimal scatter, and a well-defined radiation treatment beam.[16,52,53,54] Specifically, the fall-off of the radiation dose along the lateral edges of the treatment beam is from 90% to 50% of the total dose within 1.5 mm.[52] Charged particle radiation travels through tissue in a nearly straight line and stops after a certain distance, depending on the initial energy of the beam. This produces a drop-off of the radiation dose at the terminal end of the beam from 90% to 50% within approximately 2 mm.[52] Also, the density of ionization of the charged particles is higher near the end of their travel range, which produces an increase in the dose in that area. This is called the Bragg peak of

Table 9.3
Ruthenium Plaque Results

Report	Num	Tumor Size	Regression	Metastatic Death	Enucleation	Survival*
Lommatzsch F/U: 5 to 21 yrs	227	77% ≤ 15mm diam & ≤ 5 mm elev.	**Total:** 47% **Partial:** 24% **No Change:** 10%	19.4%	16.3%	88.17% 79.7%
Foerster et al. F/U: < 5 yrs	295	**Tumor height:** ≤ 3.8 mm: 32.3% > 3.8 to 7.7 mm: 50.2% > 7.7 mm: 17.5%	**Total:** 11.9% **Partial:** 75%	2%	11%	N/A†
Hallerman Mean F/U: 3 yrs	215	N/A	N/A	5%	5%	80%
Busse et al. F/U: 1 to 3 yrs	36	"Majority" < 5 mm elev.	**Total:** 66% **Partial:** 25% **No Change:** 8%	5%	3%	N/A

* Metastatic deaths only, 5 year survival, second number 10 year survival, if available.

† N/A: Not available.

ionization.[16,52] The radiation dosage is more uniform in the treatment area than can be achieved with plaque therapy (recall that with plaque radiotherapy more radiation is delivered to the base of the tumor than to the apex). These characteristics have generated particular enthusiasm for charged particle radiation treatment of tumors close to the fovea or optic nerve.[55] But treatment of more posterior tumors may require significantly more radiation exposure to anterior segment structures than plaque therapy (additional radiation exposure occurs with charged particle radiation where the external radiation beam enters the eye).[85]

The treatment dose, usually, has been 70 Cobalt Gy equivalent (CGE), though higher and lower doses have occasionally been used.[11,16,57,68] The relative biologic effectiveness (page 93) of proton beam compared with cobalt-60 irradiation is estimated to be approximately 1.1.[53] The 70 CGE treatment dose represents the actual radiation dose delivered multiplied by 1.1. The ideal radiation dose is not known, and a recent report suggests that lower doses may be as effective as higher doses.[68] Larger tumors may be more amenable to irradiation with charged particles than to brachytherapy.[15,52] A disadvantage of charged particle irradiation is the expense and limited availability of treatment facilities. Also, anterior segment complications may be more frequent than with ^{125}I plaque radiotherapy.[17]

Charged particle radiation does not avoid a surgical procedure.[24] It is necessary to surgically attach several 2.5 mm tantalum marker rings to the sclera along the edge of the tumor; this allows later radiologic determination of the tumor margins to aim the radiation beam.[10,53] Tumors confined to the ciliary body, the anterior choroid, or both, do not necessarily need placement of the clips. A computer program, using the length of the eye, the position of the clips relative to the tumor, and the position of the tumor relative to structures within the eye, allows three-dimensional viewing of the planned treatment area and permits alterations in the eye position to minimize radiation exposure to important structures.[49] Treatment is divided into four or five sessions and is given over a seven- to ten-day period.

Charged Particle Radiation Treatment Results

Signs of a treatment response are similar to brachytherapy. Resolution of an exudative retinal detachment is usually the earliest evidence of a treatment response, though occasionally an initial increase in the retinal detachment occurs.[25,55,68,119] Other signs of tumor regression include yellowish discoloration of the apical portion of the tumor, and fluorescein angiographic evidence of destruction of tumor vessels and absence of fluorescein leakage.

Table 9.4
Proton Beam Irradiation

SURVIVAL AND PROGNOSTIC FACTORS FOLLOWING PROTON BEAM IRRADIATION

	% Alive ± Standard Error			
	1 Year	2 Years	3 Years	4 Years
Largest Diameter				
< 10.0 mm	100	99 ± 1	97 ± 2	97 ± 2
10.1 to 15.0 mm	98 ± 1	96 ± 1	94 ± 2	91 ± 4
> 15 mm	91 ± 2	84 ± 3	76 ± 5	69 ± 7
Tumor Location				
Posterior	99 ± 1	98 ± 1	98 ± 2	96 ± 2
Anterior	96 ± 1	91 ± 3	88 ± 4	85 ± 6
Ciliary Body	89 ± 2	82 ± 4	72 ± 5	64 ± 8
Age (Years)				
< 59	98 ± 1	95 ± 1	92 ± 2	88 ± 3
> 59	93 ± 1	88 ± 2	83 ± 4	81 ± 5
Extrascleral Extension				
No	96 ± 1	93 ± 1	89 ± 2	86 ± 3
Yes	78 ± 9	61 ± 14	49 ± 17	49 ± 17

From Gragoudas ES, Seddon JM, Egan KM, et al.: Metastasis from uveal melanoma after proton beam irradiation. Ophthalmology 95:992-999, 1988.

Local tumor control (defined as a decrease in tumor size or no continued growth) occurs in approximately 98% of cases.[55,68] As with plaque therapy, tumors did not regress for six months or longer following treatment. Complete regression to a flat scar is unusual and occurs in only 12% of eyes.[55]

Metastatic disease has developed in 8% to 12% of treated patients.[57,68] But only about 30% of the patients in these reports have been followed for three or more years. The five-year cumulative probability of metastasis following proton beam therapy was calculated as 20%.[57] Metastases were detected from three months up to 7.3 years after treatment. The annual rate of metastasis was 1.4% (year 1), 3.7% (year 2), 5.0%(year 3), 5.3% (year 4), 5.9%(year 5) and 4.1% (years 6-8).

Prognostic factors for developing metastatic melanoma following charged particle therapy are similar to those in patients undergoing enucleation.[56,57,68] Important factors are the largest diameter of the tumor (tumors > 15 mm in diameter: worse prognosis), location of the anterior margin of the tumor anterior to the equator, tumor height, the age of the patient at time of treatment (age over 59 had less favorable prognosis), and presence of extrascleral extension.[57,68] The calculated four-year survival for some of these categories is shown in **Table 9.4** (above). Local recurrence of melanoma did not appear to be a poor prognostic factor.

A recent study evaluated rate of tumor regression as a prognostic factor.[51] When pretreatment risk characteristics were statistically controlled, more rapid tumor regression during the first two years following proton beam irradiation was associated with a higher risk of metastasis during this two-year period. Interestingly, a slower rate of tumor regression two or more years following treatment was associated with a higher risk of metastasis two or more years following treatment. Additionally, pretreatment characteristics such as age at the time of diagnosis and ciliary body involvement were not significant prognostic factors for metastasis two or more years following treatment.[51]

The treatment of malignant melanoma with ciliary body involvement is difficult because of the potential for radiation damage to the anterior segment. Resection of medium-sized and smaller tumors is possible, but larger tumors are less amenable to this approach. Results of treatment of ciliochoroidal tumors with proton or helium ion therapy suggest that many can be successfully treated and the eye retained. Follow-up in two reported series is short, but 75% to 90% of patients have retained their eye, although multiple complications due to the tumor or radiation treatment were noted, and most lost vision.[11,14]

Enucleation of treated eyes has been necessary for complications from radiation and also inadequate tumor control in approximately 6% to 11% of treated patients.[25,55] The most serious complication has been rubeosis irides and neovascular glaucoma, which has occurred in 13% to 15% of proton and helium ion treated eyes.[55,66] This occurs more frequently following treatment of larger tumors and eyes that receive more anterior segment or total irradiation.[55,66] The location of the tumor does not appear to be a significant risk factor. Other complications have included radiation retinopathy or optic neuropathy (15% to 20%), cataracts (7% to 43%), lash loss or lid erythema (61%), vitreous hemorrhage (1%), punctal occlusion (1%), and retinal neovascularization (2%).[25,55] Recently, one case of sympathetic ophthalmia was diagnosed approximately four years following helium ion radiation treatment of a choroidal melanoma.[44]

Table 9.5
Proton Beam Irradiation

	CUMULATIVE PERCENT RETAINING VISION 20/200 OR BETTER		
Risk Group*	1 Year	2 Years	3 Years
Good	100	96 ± 4	91 ± 7
Fair	84 ± 3[†]	68 ± 4	61 ± 6
Poor	51 ± 5	33 ± 7	24 ± 7

Risk Groups:*

Good: Tumor height ≤ 5 mm
Tumor > 2 disc-diameters from fovea and optic nerve
Pretreatment visual acuity > 20/40

Fair: Tumor height > 5 mm OR tumor within 2 disc-diameters
of fovea and/or optic nerve.

Poor: Tumor height > 5 mm AND tumor within 2 disc-diameters
of fovea and/or optic nerve

[†] Percent ± standard deviation.
From Seddon JM, Gragoudas ES, Polivogianis L, Hsieh CC, et al.: Visual outcome
after proton beam irradiation of uveal melanoma. Ophthalmology 93:666-674, 1986.

Visual acuity results depend on the length of follow-up (radiation retinopathy may take several years to develop); the position and size of the tumor; the presence or absence of macular detachment; the amount of radiation to the fovea, disc, or lens; and the pretreatment visual acuity.[107] Specifically, a worse prognosis for good vision following proton beam radiation therapy is associated with a pretreatment visual acuity of 20/40 or less; tumor height greater than 5 mm; tumor proximity (< 2 disc-diameters) to the fovea, the disc, or both; macular detachment; and finally, foveal and optic disc radiation dose of over 35.5 cobalt Gy equivalent.[107] **Table 9.5** (above) lists the cumulative percentage of eyes retaining a visual acuity of 20/200 or better based on the three most important prognostic factors. The leading cause of visual loss in eyes with tumors near the disc or fovea is retinal detachment. Eyes with tumors near both the optic disc and fovea have a much higher rate of visual loss below 20/200 than do eyes with tumors near the disc or fovea only.[105]

COMBINED ENUCLEATION AND RADIATION TREATMENT

Adjunct radiation therapy preceding or following surgical excision of several nonocular tumors can reduce local recurrence and mortality.[48,93,94] This approach has been applied to malignant melanomas in nonrandomized studies.[16,22,23,101] Retrospective studies have shown no reduction, or some reduction in mortality in patients treated with up to 60 Gy (6000 rads) following enucleation.[65,70,95]

An alternative approach is radiation treatment preceding enucleation.[16] Adjunctive radiation therapy prior to enucleation is considered particularly attractive in view of concern of possible tumor cell dissemination at the time of enucleation.[122] The rationale for this approach is to achieve at least partial tumor cell inactivation before surgical manipulation.[94] Relatively low doses of radiation can inactivate most tumor cells. Therefore, if tissue handling and ocular manipulations during enucleation can cause spread of tumor cells, preoperative radiation may enhance survival. The possible benefit of radiation treatment prior to enucleation is currently being investigated in the Collaborative Ocular Melanoma Study.[116]

Limitations of treatment include nonoptimal radiation dosage and the possibility of micrometastasis that might have occurred before diagnosis and treatment of the melanoma.[22,93,94] Experimental evidence, however, has suggested a possible benefit to this approach.[3,42,102] In a mouse and a Greene melanoma hamster model pre-enucleation radiation produced longer survival than that of the control group.[42,102] Additionally, radiation doses of 10 Gy to 20 Gy (1000 to 2000 rads) reduces DNA synthesis in experimental models,[102] reduces the ability of experimental tumor cells to establish metastatic foci,[102] decreases in vitro cell growth and viability of human malignant melanoma cells,[23,63,101] and reduces human melanoma tumor mitotic activity.[3,19,82]

In a nonrandomized series, 41 patients received 20 Gy (2000 rads) in five divided 4 Gy fractions before enucleation.[23] Comparison with a historical control group showed a more rapid onset of metastatic death in the irradiated group that is unexpected and difficult to explain. It seems unlikely that pre-enucleation irradiation would produce a more rapid incidence of metastasis and further investigation is necessary.[30]

The benefit, or lack of benefit, of irradiation preceding enucleation is not known and ultimately requires assessment with a randomized, clinical trial. In the Collaborative Ocular Melanoma Study, patients with large tumors (larger than 16 mm basal diameter or 8 mm in elevation) are randomized to standard enucleation, or enucleation preceded with 20 Gy (2000 rads) of irradiation (in five daily fractions of 4 Gy). The results of this study should resolve whether the use of pre-enucleation radiation therapy is beneficial.

ENUCLEATION COMPARED WITH RADIATION THERAPY

Enucleation and radiation therapy are the most commonly used methods to treat malignant melanoma. No randomized prospective data are currently available to indicate which treatment produces higher patient survival. The Collaborative Ocular Melanoma Study was planned and begun to answer this fundamental question. This prospective study randomizes patients with medium-sized tumors (2.5 mm to 10 mm in height, basal diameter up to 16 mm) for treatment with ^{125}I plaque therapy or enucleation.

The issue of survival following enucleation compared with survival following radiation treatment has been investigated in five published retrospective studies.[2,4,47,104,106] (See **Table 9.6**.) One such evaluation was by Kiehl and associates.[64] Their series, encompassing a country-wide effort in the German Democratic Republic, comprised 1,419 patients from 10 centers during a 20-year period. Approximately 16% were managed by ruthenium plaque therapy and 84% underwent enucleation. Life table analysis of survival compared radiation and enucleation treatment among those eyes with small tumors (defined as less than 10 mm × 10 mm × 2 mm) and survival following radiation or enucleation treatment among those eyes with large tumors (defined as larger than 10 mm × 10 mm × 2 mm). Deaths from all causes were reported. The 10-year survival for patients with small tumors treated with a ruthenium plaque was 72% and 49% for those patients in the enucleated group.

In 1985, Gass reported a comparison of 27 patients who underwent enucleation with 21 patients who underwent ^{60}Co plaque therapy.[47] Follow-up was for a minimum of five years. The five-year survival from metastatic death was 50% in the cobalt plaque group and 84% in the enucleation group. This is the only study that has demonstrated a treatment benefit for enucleation. But Gass noted that the cobalt plaque treated group had more tumors in an anterior location. Gamel subsequently performed a Cox regression statistical analysis that took this difference into account, and could not demonstrate a statistically significant relationship between survival and treatment modality.[45]

Seddon and associates, in 1985, compared 120 patients treated with proton beam therapy with one group of 235 patients and a second group of 161 patients who underwent enucleation

Table 9.6
Enucleation Compared with Radiation Therapy

| Report | Number | SURVIVAL | |
		Enucleation	Radiation
Kiehl et al.[64]	1,419	49%[*]	72%
Gass[47]	48	84%[†]	50%
Seddon et al.[104]	516	82%[‡,§] 90%[‡,§]	96%
Seddon et al.[106]	1051	74%[†,§] 68%[†,§]	81%[†]
Adams et al.[2]	639	Not available	Not available
Augsburger et al.[4]	237	64%[†]	74%[†]

[*] 10 year survival.

[†] 5 year survival.

[‡] 3 year survival.

[§] Two different enucleation groups taken from different and nonoverlapping time periods.

All survival figures listed are not adjusted for different tumor and patient characteristics.

between 1953 to 1973 and 1975 to 1981, respectively.[104] Survival from metastatic disease was significantly better in the proton beam treated eyes compared with the enucleation group treated between 1953 and 1973. A reduced difference in survival was present when the more recent enucleation group was compared with the proton beam group.

Augsburger and associates compared 237 patients undergoing enucleation with 97 patients undergoing cobalt plaque therapy; there was a minimum of 3.5 years follow-up.[4] Adjustment for differences in patient and tumor characteristics within the enucleation and radiation treatment group revealed no statistically significant difference between these treatment modalities.

More recently, Adams and associates compared 223 patients treated with cobalt-60 plaques with 416 patients who underwent enucleation; patient statistics were obtained from several centers.[2] In this study also, no statistically significant difference between these treatment groups was noted.

Seddon and her co-workers recently reported a series of 556 patients treated with proton beam irradiation with 238 patients treated with enucleation during the same period, and 257 patients enucleated during the preceding 10 years.[106] These authors again concluded that the type of treatment was not a significant factor in determining patient prognosis.

In evaluating any retrospective analysis, despite careful use of statistics to control for known factors that may influence results, uncontrolled biases may influence results.[4,37,99,104,106] Moreover, an evaluation of one of these studies demonstrated that the 95% confidence intervals were large enough such that the true mortality in either treatment group could be as much as twice that of the other treatment group.[4,37,99] Therefore, which treatment is most ideal is not clear. Some authorities strongly believe that enucleation is preferable because radiation therapy is not a proven treatment due to limited follow-up information.[79] Alternatively, radiation treatment has many advocates. At this time no definitive data exists to conclude which form of treatment is best in terms of patient survival.

REFERENCES

1. Abramson DH, Servodidio, CA, McCormick B, et al.: Changes in height of choroidal melanomas after plaque therapy. Br J Ophthalmol 74:359-362, 1990.

2. Adams KS, Abramson DH, Ellsworth RM, et al.: Cobalt plaque versus enucleation for uveal melanoma: Comparison of survival rates. Br J Ophthalmol 72:494-497, 1988.

3. Augsburger JJ, Eagle RC, Chiu M, Shields JA: The effect of pre-enucleation radiotherapy on mitotic activity of choroidal and ciliary body melanomas. Ophthalmology 94:1627-1630, 1987.

4. Augsburger JJ, Gamel JW, Sardi VF, et al.: Enucleation vs. cobalt plaque radiotherapy for malignant melanomas of the choroid and ciliary body. Arch Ophthalmol 104:655-661, 1986.

5. Augsburger JJ, Gamel JW, Shields JA, et al.: Post-irradiation regression of choroidal melanomas as a risk factor for death from metastatic disease. Ophthalmology 94:1173-1177, 1987.

6. Augsburger JJ, Gonder JR, Amsel J, et al.: Growth rates and doubling times of posterior uveal melanomas. Ophthalmology 91:1709-1715, 1984.

7. Augsburger JJ, McNeary BT, von Below H, et al.: Regression of posterior uveal malignant melanomas after cobalt plaque radiotherapy. Graefe's Arch Clin Exp Ophthal 224:397-400, 1986.

8. Bedford MA: The use and abuse of cobalt plaques in the treatment of choroidal malignant melanomata. Tr Ophthalmol Soc UK 93:139-143, 1973.

9. Boniuk NM, Cohen JS: Combined use of radiation plaques and photocoagulation in the treatment of choroidal melanomas. In Jakobiec F. (Ed): Ocular and Adnexal Tumors. Birmingham, Aesculapius Company, 1978, pp 80-88.

10. Brockhurst RJ: Tantalum buttons for localization of malignant melanoma in proton beam therapy. Ophthalmic Surg 11:352, 1980.

11. Brovkina AF, Zarubei GD: Ciliochoroidal melanomas treated with a narrow medical proton beam. Arch Ophthalmol 104:402-404, 1986.

12. Busse H, Muller RP: Techniques and results of 106Ru/106Rh radiation of choroidal tumours. Tr Ophthalmol Soc UK 103:72-77, 1983.

13. Busse H, Muller RP, Kroll P: Results of 106-Ru/Rh radiation of choroidal melanomas. Ann Ophthalmol 15:1146-1149, 1983.

14. Char DH: Radiation therapy for uveal melanomas involving the ciliary body. Tr Ophthalmol Soc UK 105:252-256, 1986.

15. Char DH: Clinical Ocular Oncology. New York, Churchill Livingstone, 1989, pp 91-149.

16. Char DH, Castro JR: Helium ion therapy for choroidal melanoma. Arch Ophthalmol 100:935-938, 1982.

17. Char DH, Castro JR, Quivey JM, et al.: Uveal melanoma radiation. ^{125}I brachytherapy versus helium ion irradiation. Ophthalmol 96:1708-1715, 1989.

18. Char DH, Crawford JB, Castro JR, Woodruff KH: Failure of choroidal melanoma to respond to helium ion therapy. Arch Ophthalmol 101:236-241, 1983.

19. Char DH, Huhta K, Waldman F: DNA Cell cycle studies in uveal melanoma. Am J Ophthalmol 107:65-72, 1989.

20. Char DH, Lonn LI, Margolis LW: Complications of cobalt plaque therapy of choroidal melanomas. Am J Ophthalmol 84:536-541, 1977.

21. Char DH, Miller TR, Ljung BM, et al.: Fine needle aspiration biopsy in uveal melanoma. Presented at Advances and Controversies in the Management of Ocular and Periocular Malignancies. San Francisco, December, 1988.

22. Char DH, Phillips TL: Pre-Enucleation irradiation of uveal melanoma. Br J Ophthalmol 69:177-179, 1985.

23. Char DH, Phillips TL, Andejeski Y, et al.: Failure of preenucleation radiation to decrease uveal melanoma mortality. Am J Ophthalmol 106:21-26, 1988.

24. Char DH, Castro JR, Quivey JM, et al.: Uveal melanoma radiation. ^{125}I brachytherapy versus helium ion irradiation. Ophthalmology 96:1708-1715, 1989.

25. Char DH, Saunders W, Castro JR, et al.: Helium ion therapy for choroidal melanoma. Ophthalmology 90:1219-1225, 1983.

26. Coleman DJ, Lizzi FL, Silverman RH, et al.: Regression of uveal malignant melanomas following cobalt-60 plaque. Correlates between acoustic spectrum analysis and tumor regression. Retina 5:73-78, 1985.

27. Crawford JB, Char DH: Histopathology of uveal melanomas treated with charged particle radiation. Ophthalmology 94:639-643, 1987.

28. Cruess AF, Augsburger JJ, Shields JA, et al.: Visual results following cobalt plaque radiotherapy for posterior uveal melanomas. Ophthalmology 91:131-136, 1984.

29. Cruess AF, Augsburger JJ, Shields JA, et al.: Regression of posterior uveal melanomas following cobalt-60 plaque radiotherapy. Ophthalmology 91:1716-1719, 1984.

30. Collaborative Ocular Melanoma Study Group, Fine SL, Straatsma BR, Earle JD, et al.: Failure of preenucleation radiation to decrease uveal melanoma mortality. Letter to the editor. Am J Ophthalmol 107:440-441, 1989.

31. Davidorf FH, Pajka JT, Makley TA, Kartha MK: Radiotherapy for choroidal melanoma. An 18-year experience with radon. Arch Ophthalmol 105:352-355, 1987.

32. Duker JS, Augsburger JJ, Shields JA: Noncontiguous local recurrence of posterior uveal melanoma after cobalt 60 plaque therapy. Arch Ophthalmol 107:1019-1022, 1989.

33. Earle J, Kline RW, Robertson DM: Selection of iodine 125 for the collaborative ocular melanoma study. Arch Ophthalmol 105:763-765, 1987.

34. Ellsworth RM: The treatment of malignant melanoma of the uvea. Trans Aust Coll Ophthalmol 3:57-60, 1971.

35. Ellsworth RM: Cobalt plaques for melanoma of the choroid. In Ocular and Adnexal Tumors. Jakobiec F (Ed). Aesculapius, Birmingham, 1978, pp 76-79.

36. Ferry AP, Blair CJ, Gragoudas ES, Volk SC: Pathologic examination of ciliary body melanoma treated with proton beam irradiation. Arch Ophthalmol 103:1849-1853, 1985.

37. Fine SL: Do I take the eye out or leave it in? Arch Ophthalmol 104:653-654, 1986.

38. Fish GE, Jost BF, Snyder WB, et al.: Cataract extraction after brachytherapy for malignant melanoma of the choroid. Ophthalmol 98:619-622, 1991.

39. Flynn K, Felberg NT, Koegel A, et al.: Lymphocyte subpopulations before therapy in patients with uveal malignant melanoma. Am J Ophthalmol 101:160-163, 1986.

40. Foerster MH, Bornfeld N, Schultz V, et al.: Complications of local beta radiation of uveal melanomas. Graefes Arch Clin Exp Ophthalmol 224:336-340, 1986.

41. Foerster MH, Fried M, Wessing A, Meyer-Schwickerath G: Tumor regression and functional results in sequential ruthenium therapy and photocoagulation for choroidal melanoma. In Lommatzsch PK, Blodi FC (Eds): Intraocular Tumors. New York, Springer-Verlag, 1983, pp 316-340.

42. Fournier GA, Saulenas AM, Seddon JM, et al.: The effects of pre-enucleation irradiation on the development of metastases from intraocular Greene melanoma in hamsters. Am J Ophthalmol 100:669-677, 1985.

43. Frazier-Byrne S, Olsen KR, Houdek P, et al.: Intraoperative plaque localization with contact B-scan echography. Submitted for Publication, 1989.

44. Fries PD, Char DH, Crawford JB, Waterhouse W: Sympathetic ophthalmia complicating helium ion irradiation of a choroidal melanoma. Arch Ophthalmol 105:1561-1564, 1987.

45. Gamel JW: Ocular Melanoma. Correspondence. Arch Ophthalmol 103:1284, 1985.

46. Garretson BR, Robertson DM, Earle JD: Choroidal melanoma treatment with iodine 125 brachytherapy. Arch Ophthalmol 105:1394-1397, 1987.

47. Gass JDM: Comparison of prognosis after enucleation vs. cobalt 60 irradiation of melanomas. Arch Ophthalmol 103:916-923, 1985.

48. Glicksman AS: Combined sequential radiotherapy and surgery in the management of malignancies. Rh Isl Med J 48:538-543, 1965.

49. Goitein M, Miller T: Planning proton therapy of the eye. Med Phys 10:275-283, 1983.

50. Goodman DF, Char DH, Crawford JB, et al.: Uveal melanoma necrosis after helium ion therapy. Am J Ophthalmol 101:643-645, 1986.

51. Glynn RJ, Seddon JM, Gragoudas ES, et al.: Evaluation of tumor regresion and other prognostic factors for early and late metastasis after proton irradiation of uveal melanoma. Ophthalmology 96:1566-1573, 1989.

52. Gragoudas ES: The Bragg peak of proton beams for treatment of uveal melanoma. Int Ophthalmol Clin 20:123-133, 1980.

53. Gragoudas ES, Goitein M, Koehler A, Constable IJ, et al.: Proton irradiation of choroidal melanomas. Preliminary results. Arch Ophthalmol 96:1583-1591, 1978.

54. Gragoudas ES, Goitein M, Koehler AM, et al.: Proton irradiation of small choroidal malignant melanomas. Am J Ophthalmol 83:665-673, 1977.

55. Gragoudas ES, Seddon JM, Egan K, et al.: Long-term results of proton beam irradiated uveal melanomas. Ophthalmology 94:349-353, 1987.

56. Gragoudas ES, Seddon JM, Egan KM, et al.: Prognostic factors for metastasis following proton beam irradiation of uveal melanomas. Ophthalmology 93:675-680, 1986.

57. Gragoudas ES, Seddon JM, Egan KM, et al.: Metastasis from uveal melanoma after proton beam irradiation. Ophthalmology 95:992-999, 1988.

58. Grizzard WS, Torczynski E, Char DH: Helium ion charged-particle therapy for choroidal melanoma. Histopathologic findings in a successfully treated case. Arch Ophthalmol 102:576-578, 1984.

59. Hall EJ: Radiobiology for the radiologist. Philadelphia, JB Lippincott, 1988, pp 27-35, 138-160, 162-177, 294-329.

60. Hallerman D: Treatment of intraocular melanomas by ruthenium-106 beta irradiation. In Oosterhuis JA (Ed): Ophthalmic Tumors. Dordrecht, Junk Publishers, 1985, pp 55-75.

61. Kaplan HJ: Lymphocyte subpopulations in uveal malignant melanoma. Am J Ophthalmol 101:483-485, 1986.

62. Karlsson UL, Augsburger JJ, Shields JA, et al.: Recurrence of posterior uveal melanoma after ^{60}cobalt episcleral plaque therapy. Ophthalmology 96:382-388, 1989.

63. Kenneally CZ, Farber MG, Smith ME, Devineni R: In vitro melanoma cell growth after preenucleation radiation therapy. Arch Ophthalmol 106:223-224, 1988.

64. Kiehl H, Kirsch I: Treatment of malignant choroidal melanomas: Comparison of survival after conservative (^{106}Ru/^{106}Rh applicator) treatment and enucleation, first results of a GDR-wide study, 1960-1980. In Lommatzsch PK, Blodi FC (Eds): Intraocular Tumors. New York, Springer-Verlag, 1983, pp 109-112.

65. Kiehl H, Kirsch I, Lommatzsch P: Survival after treatment for malignant choroidal melanoma: Comparison between conservative therapy (^{106}Ru/^{106}Rh applicator) and enucleation with and without postoperative irradiation. Klin Mbl Augenheilk 184:2-14, 1984.

66. Kim MK, Char DH, Castro JL, et al.: Neovascular glaucoma after helium ion irradiation for uveal melanoma. Ophthalmology 93:189-193, 1986.

67. Kincaid MC, Folberg R, Torczynski E, et al.: Complications after proton beam therapy for uveal malignant melanoma. A clinical and histopathologic study of five cases. Ophthalmology 95:982-991, 1988.

68. Kindy-Degnan NA, Char DH, Castro JR, et al.: Effect of various doses of radiation for uveal melanoma on regression, visual acuity, complications, and survival. Am J Ophthalmol 107:114-120, 1989.

69. Lommatzsch P: B-Irradiation of choroidal melanoma with ^{106}Ru/^{106}Rh applicators. Sixteen years' experience. Arch Ophthalmol 101:713, 1983.

70. Lommatzsch P, Dietrich B: The effect of orbital irradiation on the survival rate of patients with choroidal melanoma. Ophthalmologica 173:49-52, 1976.

71. Lommatzsch PK: Treatment of choroidal melanomas with Ru-106/Rh-106 beta-ray applicators. Surv Ophthalmol 19:85-100, 1074.

72. Lommatzsch PK: Results after B-irradiation (^{106}Ru/^{106}Rh) of choroidal melanomas: 20 years experience. Br J Ophthalmol 70:844-851, 1986.

73. Lommatzsch PK, Kirsch IH: ^{106}Ru/^{106}Rh plaque radiotherapy for malignant melanomas of the choroid. With follow-up results more than 5 years. Doc Ophthalmol 68:225-238, 1988.

74. Long RS, Galin MA, Rotman M: Conservative treatment of intraocular melanomas. Tr Am Acad Ophthalmol Oto 75:84-93, 1971.

75. MacFaul PA: Local radiotherapy in the treatment of malignant melanoma of the choroid. Tr Ophthalmol Soc UK 97:421-427, 1977.

76. MacFaul PA: The place of radiotherapy in the treatment of uveal melanoma. Doc Ophthalmol 50:63-69, 1980.

77. MacFaul PA, Morgan G: Histopathological changes in malignant melanoma of the choroid after cobalt plaque therapy. Br J Ophthalmol 61:221-228, 1977.

78. Malbran E, Dodds R, D'Allessandro C: Conservative treatment of uveal melanomas. Mod Probl Ophthalmol 12:567-575, 1974.

79. Manschot WA, Van Strik R: Is irradiation a justifiable treatment of choroidal melanoma? Analysis of published results. Br J Ophthalmol 71:348-352, 1987.

80. Migdal C: Choroidal melanoma: The role of conservative therapy. Tr Ophthalmol Soc UK 103:54-58, 1983.

81. Moore RF: Choroidal sarcoma treated by the intraocular insertion of radon seeds. Br J Ophthalmol 14:145-152, 1930.

82. Mooy CM, de Jong PT, Van der Kwast TH, et al.: Ki-67 immunostaining in uveal melanoma. Ophthalmology 97:1275-1280, 1990.

83. Moura RA, McPherson AR, Easley J: Malignant melanoma of the choroid: Treatment with episcleral ^{198}Au plaque and xenon-arc photocoagulation. Ann Ophthalmol 17:114-125, 1985.

84. Newman GH, Davidorf FH, Havener WH, Makley TA: Conservative management of malignant melanoma. I. Irradiation as a method of treatment for malignant melanoma of the choroid. Arch Ophthalmol 83:21-26, 1970.

85. Packer S: Iodine-125 radiation of posterior uveal melanoma. Ophthalmology 94:1621-1626, 1987.

86. Packer S, Fairchild RG, Salanitro P: New techniques for iodine-125 radiotherapy of intraocular tumors. Ann Ophthalmol 19:26-30, 1987.

87. Packer S, Rotman M: Radiotherapy of choroidal melanoma with iodine 125. Int Ophthalmol Clin 20:135-142, 1980.

88. Packer S, Rotman M, Salanitro P: Iodine-125 irradiation of choroidal melanoma. Clinical experience. Ophthalmology 91:1700-1708, 1984.

89. Packer S, Rotman M: Radiotherapy of choroidal melanoma with iodine-125. Ophthalmology 87:582-590, 1980.

90. Pavlin CJ, Japp B, Payne DG, et al.: Intraoperative use of ultrasound in the management of choroidal melanomas. In Ossoinig KC (Ed): Ophthalmic Echography, The Netherlands, Nijhoff-Junk, 1987, pp 391-399.

91. Pavlin CJ, Japp B, Simpson R, et al.: Ultrasound determination of the relationship of radioactive plaques to the base of choroidal melanomas. Ophthalmology 96:538-542, 1989.

92. Polivogianis L, Seddon JM, Glynn RJ, et al.: Comparision of transillumination and histologic slide measurements of tumor diameter in uveal melanoma. Ophthalmology 95:1576-1582, 1988.

93. Powers WE, Tolmach LJ: Preoperative radiation therapy: Biological basis and experimental investigations. Nature 201:272-273, 1964.

94. Powers WE, Palmer LA: Biologic basis of preoperative radiation treatment. Am J Roentgenology 102:176-192, 1968.

95. Raivio I: Uveal melanoma in Finland. An epidemiological, clinical, histological and prognostic study. Acta Ophthalmol 133:5-64, 1977.

96. Robertson DM, Earle J, Anderson JA: Preliminary observations regarding the use of iodine-125 in the management of choroidal melanoma. Tr Ophthalmol Soc UK 103:155-160, 1983.

97. Robertson DM, Fountain KS, Anderson AJ, Posthumus GW: Radioactive iodine-125 as a therapeutic radiation source for management of intraocular tumors. Tr Am Ophthalmol Soc 79:294-306, 1981.

98. Robertson DM, Fuller DG, Anderson RE: A technique for accurate placement of episcleral iodine-125 plaques. Am J Ophthalmol 103:63-65, 1987.

99. Robertson DM: A rationale for comparing radiation to enucleation in the management of choroidal melanoma. Editorial. Am J Ophthalmol 108:448-451, 1989.

100. Rotman M, Long RS, Packer S, et al.: Radiation therapy of choroidal melanoma. Tr Ophthalmol Soc UK 97:431-435, 1977.

101. Rousseau A, Boudreault G, Deschenes J: Malignant melanoma. Radiation therapy prior to enucleation. In Henkind P. (Ed): Acta XIIII, International Congress of Ophthalmology. Philiadelphia, Lippincott, 1983, pp 983-987.

102. Sanborn GE, Ngyuen P, Gamel J, Niederkorn JY: Reduction of enucleation-induced metastasis in intraocular melanoma by periorbital irradiation. Arch Ophthalmol 105:1260-1264, 1987.

103. Seddon JM, Gragoudas ES, Albert DM: Ciliary body and choroidal melanomas treated by proton beam irradiation. Histopathologic study of eyes. Arch Ophthalmol 101:1402-1408, 1983.

104. Seddon JM, Gragoudas ES, Albert DM, et al.: Comparison of survival rates for patients with uveal melanoma after treatment with proton beam irradiation or enucleation. Am J Ophthalmol 99:282-290, 1985.

105. Seddon JM, Gragoudas ES, Egan KM, et al.: Uveal melanomas near the optic disc or fovea. Visual results after proton beam irradiation. Ophthalmology 94:354-361, 1987.

106. Seddon JM, Gragoudas ES, Egan KM, et al.: Relative survival rates after alternative therapies for uveal melanoma. Ophthalmology 97:769-777, 1990.

107. Seddon JM, Gragoudas ES, Polivogianis L, et al.: Visual outcome after proton beam irradiation of uveal melanoma. Ophthalmology 93:666-674, 1986.

108. Shields CL, Shields JA, Karlsson U, et al.: Reasons for enucleation after plaque radiotherapy for posterior uveal melanoma. Clinical findings. Ophthalmology 96:919-924, 1989.

109. Shields CL, Shields JA, Karlsson U, et al.: Enucleation after plaque radiotherapy for posterior uveal melanoma. Histopathologic findings. Ophthalmology 97:1665-1670, 1990.

110. Shields JA, Augsburger JJ, Brady LW, Day JL: Cobalt plaque therapy of posterior uveal melanomas. Ophthalmology 89:1201-1207, 1982.

111. Stallard HB: Radiotherapy for malignant melanoma of the choroid. Br J Ophthalmol 50:147-155, 1966.

112. Stallard HB: Radiant energy as (a) a pathogenic, (b) a therapeutic agent in ophthalmic disorders. Br J Ophthalmol Monograph (Suppl, 1933.

113. Stallard HB: Radiotherapy of malignant intra-ocular neoplasms. Br J Ophthalmol 32:618-639, 1948.

114. Stallard HB: Comparative value of radium and deep x-rays in the treatment of retinoblastoma. Br J Ophthalmol 36:313-324, 1952.

115. Stallard HB: Malignant melanoblastoma of the choroid. Mod Probl Ophthalmol 7:16-38, 1968.

116. Straatsma BR, Fine SL, Earle JD, et al.: Enucleation versus plaque irradiation for choroidal melanoma. Ophthalmology 95:1000-1004, 1988.

117. Tsukerman M, Barishak YR: The effect of conservative treatment on the choroidal melanoma: Histopathologic study. Ann Ophthalmol 10:316-321, 1978.

118. Wessing A, Foerster M, Bornfield N: Ruthenium plaque treatment of malignant choroidal melanomas. In Oosterhuis JA (Ed): Ophthalmic Tumors. Dordrecht, Junk Publishers, 1985, pp 71-85.

119. Wilkes SR, Gragoudas ES: Regression patterns of uveal melanomas after proton beam irradiation. Ophthalmology 89:840-844, 1982.

120. Williams DF, Mieler WF, Lewandowski M, Greenberg M: Echographic verification of radioactive plaque position in the treatment of melanomas. Arch Ophthalmol 106:1623-1624, 1988.

121. Withers HR, Peters LT: Biologic aspects of radiation therapy. In Fletcher GH (Ed): Textbook of Radiotherapy. Philadelphia, Lea & Febiger Publishers, 1980, pp 103-122, 153-156.

122. Zimmerman LE, McLean IW: An evaluation of enucleation in the management of uveal melanomas. Am J Ophthalmol 87:741-760, 1979.

123. Zinn KM, Stein-Pokorny K, Jakobiec FA, et al.: Proton beam irradiated epitheloid cell melanoma of the ciliary body. Ophthalmology 88:1315-1321, 1981.

124. Zografos L, Gailloud CL: Conservative treatment of choroidal melanoma by cobalt 60 applicators. In Lommatzsch PK, Blodi FC (Eds): Intraocular Tumors. New York, Springer-Verlag, 1983, pp 286-289.

125. Zografos L, Gailloud C: Cobalt plaque treatment of choroidal melanomas. In Oosterhuis JA (Ed): Ophthalmic Tumors. Dordrecht, Junk Publishers, 1985, pp 87-92.

126. Zografos L, Perret C, Gailloud C: I-125 plaque irradiation. Letter to the editor. Ophthalmology 95:1155, 1988.

127. Zygulska-Mach H, Maciejewski Z, Link, E: Conservative treatment of choroidal melanomas. Combined use of cobalt plaques and photocoagulation. In Lommatzsch PK, Blodi FC (Eds): Intraocular Tumors. New York, Springer-Verlag, 1983, pp 417-423.

CHAPTER 10

ALTERNATIVE TREATMENT MODALITIES

HYPERTHERMIA

In recent years, attention has turned to the application of hyperthermia for treatment of malignant melanoma. Hyperthermia alone has produced complete tumor regression and focal thermotoxic tissue damage in a Greene melanoma rabbit model.[9,41,73] Generally, though, hyperthermia is combined with radiation therapy; the goal of combined treatment is to reduce the required radiation dosage, thereby, theoretically minimizing complications.[12] This combined approach can achieve synergistic tissue effects.[18,37,86] Hypoxic cells are somewhat radioresistant whereas they remain sensitive to heat.[18,40,86] Radiosensitivity relates to cell cycle; cells in the S phase are radioresistant but are most sensitive to heat.[18,61,86] In general, tumor cells are more thermal sensitive. Hyperthermic treatments can be clinically performed using ultrasound,[12,13,49] electromagnetic radiation (microwaves[22,23,42] and radiofrequency[4]), and ferromagnetic thermoseeds.[57]

One method for combined therapy incorporates a microwave applicator within an ^{125}I plaque.[23,42,61] Another combined therapeutic approach incorporates ferromagnetic thermoseeds within an ^{125}I plaque.[57] Good tumor regression using this combined approach with a Greene melanoma rabbit model has been shown.[23,57] In another experimental study, a subtherapeutic dose of combined proton beam radiation and ultrasonically-induced hyperthermia produced synergistic tumor regression in most cases.[73]

Preliminary treatment results of four patients treated with several hyperthermia treatments (to about 43° C) combined with cobalt-60 plaque therapy (about 6500 rads to the apex) in three eyes and teletherapy in one eye (3900 rads), showed good tumor regression in all four, and essentially stable visual acuities.[12] Histologic studies of human eyes treated with hyperthermia (treatment temperatures to 45° C) before enucleation have shown extensive tumor damage with some perivascular sparing, presumably because of a "heat-sink" effect provided by blood flow.[13,37] Also, the inner tumor surface showed less thermal damage. Treatment temperatures of over 50° C produced more extensive damage; this suggests a possible method of tumor "sterilization" before enucleation, analogous to the rationale of external beam radiotherapy prior to enucleation.

Clinical data are very limited and preliminary. At this time, any benefit of hyperthermia as an adjunct to radiation treatment, although theoretically attractive, remains unproved. More studies evaluating treatment temperatures, fractionation, and radiation dosage are necessary.

PHOTOCOAGULATION

The use of photocoagulation for ablation of choroidal malignant melanomas was first described by Meyer-Schwickerath in 1957.[53] This procedure initially used the xenon arc photocoagulator, though today other wavelengths are used, such as krypton red and argon blue-green.[11,27,78–80]

Published criteria for treatment have included both size and fundus location. Meyer-Schwickerath and Vogel limit treatment to tumors less than 2 mm in elevation,[56,90] but others consider elevations of 3.5 mm to 4.0 mm to be the upper limit.[11,27,29] The diameter should be less than 8 mm to 10 mm.[11,29,90] Because treatment is placed around the tumor, juxtapapillary tumors are less suitable.[79,90] Also, macular tumors are less amenable to treatment because numerous short posterior ciliary arteries in this region not only increase the difficulty of ablating the tumor's blood supply but also provide more channels for extrascleral extension.[11,88,90] Retinal detachment, poor pupil dilation, and media opacities preclude treatment, as do tumors located anterior to the equator where surrounding the tumor with photocoagulation treatment may be difficult.[28,88,90] Photocoagulation treatment close to large retinal vessels may cause retinal vascular occlusion and concomitant risk of neovascularization.[90] These selective criteria have evolved after careful review of previous treatment experiences that demonstrated poor results with larger tumors located in less advantageous locations.[29,55,56,90] In one oncology center, only about 5% of cases are considered eligible for photocoagulation treatment.[11]

Detailed descriptions of photocoagulation treatment technique are well reported in the literature.[11,29,52,56,79,88,90] The treatment is divided into several sessions, typically separated by several weeks. Photocoagulation is initially performed around the tumor. The purpose of the initial surrounding treatments is to close or to decrease the tumor's blood supply and is of tantamount importance.[52,88] During subsequent treatment sessions, photocoagulation directly over the tumor mass is done (**Fig. 10.1**). Most tumors amenable to treatment require four to six treatment sessions.[11,29,55,90]

Reported results confirm that many of these tumors can be locally controlled; chances of success correlate with the size of the tumor.[11,30,31,54] Success can be defined as an ophthalmoscopic appearance of extensive chorioretinal atrophy around the tumor margin, "bare sclera," and a mostly flat, centrally pigmented scar that remains stable.[56,88,90] Resorption of this central pigment occurs slowly and may take several years.[30,31,52] Ultrasound studies have confirmed that the scar is flat in most cases.[82] Fluorescein angiography that shows hypofluorescence of the central pigmented mass confirms ablation of the tumor's blood supply and thus the adequacy of treatment.[33] A recurrence may be suggested if new blood vessels develop within the tumor. But some consider fluorescein angiography less helpful in assessing treatment response;[90] certainly residual pigment may block fluorescence from still perfused tumor vessels.

Photocoagulation treatment can produce a local cure in up to 86% of cases.[17,30,32,48,51,54,80,91] Some smaller series with shorter follow-up have described even higher success rates.[27,72] Metastatic deaths have occurred in about 10% to 15% of treated patients. Tumor recurrence occurs in 12% to 18% of patients and can be mananged with additional laser treatment or enucleation.[17,30]

Overall, 25% to 59% of eyes have been enucleated because of recurrence or treatment complications.[17,30,54,91]

Xenon arc photocoagulation has been traditionally used for treatment of choroidal melanoma, but other current alternatives include wavelengths such as argon blue-green or krypton red. A review of 38 eyes treated for choroidal melanoma with either xenon arc or argon laser photocoagulation showed that xenon arc photocoagulation was substanially more successful in achieving tumor control (86%) than was argon laser photocoagulation (47%).[80] The reason for this large difference is not clear, but it likely reflects the known poorer penetration of the choroidal layers by the argon blue-green wavelength than by the xenon arc photocoagulator.

Visual loss following photocoagulation is common and can occur from both direct and indirect effects. A posteriorly located tumor may necessitate direct photocoagulation of the macula. Alternatively, macular edema (**Fig. 10.1B**) or macular distortion because of photocoagulation-induced traction may limit vision.[91] Unfortunately, many reports do not provide complete visual acuity data. Visual acuity results are usually best for midperipheral, nasal tumors.

Criticisms of photocoagulation treatment of malignant melanoma include concern about undetected extraocular tumor extension before treatment or following treatment if the deepest layers of the tumor are not destroyed.[55,89] Extraocular tumor extension has been found in 7% to 35% of *enucleated* globes following photocoagulation.[17,20,32,47,54,89] The exact frequency of extraocular tumor extension is not known since all treated eyes

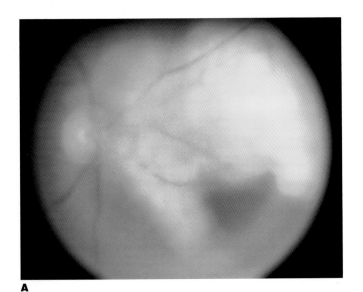
A

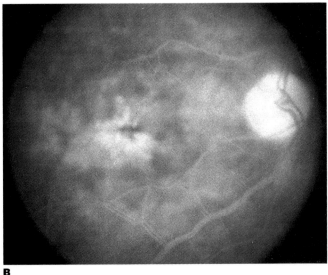
B

Figure 10.1A & B Laser Photocoagulation Of Malignant Melanoma
This 65 year-old female was noted to have an enlarging nasal peripapillary lesion that measured 11 mm × 11 mm in diameter and was 3.4 mm elevated. Intense laser photocoagulation was delivered to the surface of the tumor (Figure 10.1A). Note the small preretinal hemorrhage inferiorly. Six months later, the vision was reduced secondary to cystoid macular edema (Figure 10.1B).

have not been examined histopathologically. Tumors have recurred, usually along the treatment edge, as long as 16 years following treatment.[5,30,34] This is more common with a large tumor or one that is in a less favorable location such as adjacent to the disc.[30,34,90] Other complications include vitreous hemorrhage during or following treatment, choroido-retinal neovascularization, macular distortion from contracting scar tissue, transient exudative detachment, retinal tear and rhegmatogenous retinal detachment, iris atrophy, and uveitis.[11,20,28,30,79,88]

Histopathologic examination of eyes enucleated for various reasons following photocoagulation has demonstrated that many eyes contain viable appearing tumor cells.[5,17,38,46,47,48,52,90,91] Some have commented that the penetration of the photocoagulation effect is limited in depth.[3,14,47] Photocoagulation penetration may be reduced by the formation of fibrous scar tissue overlying the tumor.[17,30] Other findings include pigment dispersion into the vitreous. This frequently occurs during intense and direct treatment of the tumor mass; an explosive type of energy absorption may occur and produce gas bubbles, an audible pop and rupture of pigment into the vitreous.[11,52,74,90] Although some feel such vaporization of the tumor is an essential part of the photocoagulation therapy, others feel it should be avoided because of concern that dispersed loose pigment debris may result in intraocular inflammation or rupture of Bruch's membrane may provide a portal for tumor cell dissemination. Histologic examination of this pigment has not demonstrated viable tumor cells but instead has shown pigment engulfed by macrophages.[89] Histologic examination has shown closure or ablation of the tumor's blood supply.[38,46,47,89] Many of the discrepancies in reported histologic findings may be explained by histopathologic examination after only one photocoagulation treatment session compared with multiple treatments in other reports. Despite the somewhat small size of most photocoagulated tumors, many eyes respond inadequately to treatment or develop complications that severely affect visual outcome or necessitate enucleation.

Occasionally, subretinal fluid extending into the fovea **(Fig. 10.2)** is treated with less intense photocoagulation.[21] Small focal leaks can be identified with fluorescein angiography and treated specifically.[24] Alternatively, a diffuse pattern of leakage may be observed, and the entire surface of the tumor may need to be photocoagulated to treat these cases effectively.[24] Finally, subretinal neovascularization may develop over a melanocytic lesion and produce serous retinal detachment. This can be treated, with good results, with confluent and more intense treatment.[24]

PHOTORADIATION THERAPY

Photoradiation therapy (PRT) involves the administration of a photosensitizing dye, followed by low intensity light energy treatment. Light activation of this dye, most frequently

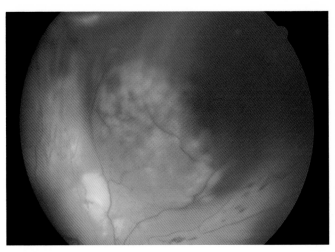

Figure 10.2 Laser Photocoagulation of Malignant Melanoma
This 63 year-old male has a 9 mm × 9 mm lesion. A serous detachment extended from the tumor to involve the fovea. Light diffuse laser photocoagulation was done.

hematoporphyrin derivative (HpD), then mediates the treatment effect.[19,76,85] An important property of HpD is its preferential uptake by tumor tissue.[19] PRT with HpD has been done for ocular and nonocular tumors. A tuneable dye laser set at 630 nm (red) maximizes tissue penetration following systemic administration of HpD.[19,77,85] The mechanisms of action are not known fully but thermal damage is not a complete explanation since the temperature elevation associated with the laser treatment in experimental systems is low,[60,76] and laser light exposure at the intensity used for PRT does not produce an effect without prior HpD treatment.[19,76] The mechanism most likely entails direct cytotoxic effects (for example through production of singlet oxygen), as well as vascular occlusive effects.[19,76]

A theoretical advantage of this therapeutic approach is to focus more precisely and to enhance the treatment to the tumor while preserving as much surrounding tissue as possible. Treatment of nonocular pigmented tumors requires more aggressive treatment than less pigmented tumors.[19,77] Experimental work with normal eyes has similarly demonstrated that light energy absorption by pigment may diminish the treatment effect to deeper tissues.[36]

Some preliminary work with photoradiation treatment of human ocular malignant melanoma has been undertaken.[8,85] Evaluation of treatment results of five patients with choroidal or ciliary body melanomas demonstrated that low intensity laser exposures and short-term follow-up prior to enucleation resulted in little or only superficial tumor necrosis.[85] But more extensive necrosis and tumor regression was apparent when the laser intensity was higher and more time elapsed before enucleation. In a larger series, but with somewhat short-term follow-up, tumor regression occurred in 16 of 18 tumors in which adequate measurements were available.[8] No histopathologic evaluation was done.

HpD treatment always causes skin sensitivity to light exposure. Ocular complications include neovascular glaucoma,[43] reduced visual acuity, and retinal detachment.[8,43] A limiting factor in the treatment of malignant melanoma may be energy absorption by pigment as described above. Currently, data are very limited, but results suggest a possible role for HpD and PRT in malignant melanoma. Further research is necessary to define more clearly and to optimize treatment parameters.

DIATHERMY

The use of diathermy alone for treatment was originally described by Weve in 1939[92] and has been used only sparingly.[16,59] There has been concern about the possibility of extraocular tumor spread, which has been noted in eyes with an unsuspected melanoma subjected to diathermy treatment during retinal detachment surgery.[6] Although the techniques used for retinal detachment surgery differ from those used for treatment of a malignant melanoma,[16] diathermy has not been widely accepted.

LOCAL RESECTION

A procedure to remove an iridociliary body melanoma was described in the German literature in the early 1900's.[87] Stallard, in 1961, described an adaptation of these techniques that could be used for resection of a choroidal melanoma.[83] Stallard's approach made a lamellar scleral flap through which a layer of overlying sclera, the uveal tumor and a margin of uninvolved uvea were excised. The retina was left intact.[83,84]

The technique of resection has been modified in many centers. Variations that have been reported include resection of partial thickness sclera with resection of the retina overlying the tumor,[50] and resection of full-thickness sclera and replacement with a donor scleral graft[35,62,67] or dacron graft.[64] Some add the routine use of vitrectomy surgery if the retina is resected overlying the tumor.[69] Hypotensive anesthesia is believed by some to provide an advantage to minimize bleeding.[25] Clinicians vary in their use of photocoagulation or cryotherapy along the margins of the tumor several weeks prior to resection.[25,50,69,75,81]

In a series of 60 cases of malignant melanoma with some degree of ciliary body involvement treated with local resection

and follow-up of one month to 16 years, nine metastatic deaths (15%) and one orbital recurrence occurred.[15,26] The mortality rate in those patients with at least five years of follow-up was 18%. Visual acuity was finger counting or better in 72% of eyes and 6/18 or better in 32%. The most common complication was vitreous hemorrhage (40%), but other complications included retinal detachment (26%) and residual tumor (20%). Thirteen eyes (22%) were enucleated because of tumor recurrence or complications; 78% of eyes were therefore retained. Complications were more common in eyes with a tumor diameter greater than 15 mm or if the tumor involved more than one-third of the ciliary body.

In other reported series, complications include vitreous hemorrhage, cataract, retinal detachment, cystoid macular edema, macular pucker, and expulsive choroidal hemorrhage.[11,26,39] Results appear to be best for tumors less than 10 mm in size and located at or anterior to the equator,[11,39,66] although some[26] believe that resection of ciliary body tumors is associated with a poorer prognosis for visual acuity. Others assert that the globe can tolerate excisions of tumors as large as 18 mm in diameter and involving five clock-hours of pars plicata.[58]

An alternative method of resection of a melanoma is through the pars plana ("ab interno").[68,70,71] This internal approach uses a vitreous cutter to remove the tumor and has the advantage of greater control of potential operative complications such as bleeding. How great the risk of spreading tumor cells through 20-gauge sclerotomies is not known but is concerning. Initial results demonstrate that this technique may be useful when a tumor is within 2 mm to 3 mm of the optic nerve.[71] Since radiation treatment of tumors that are within 2 mm to 3 mm of the optic nerve will almost invariably result in substantial loss of vision, an alternative approach that is effective and safe is desirable.

Of primary importance in evaluating a treatment for malignant melanoma is the prognosis for life; unfortunately, not only are the data limited, but there are no randomized studies comparing local resection to any other form of therapy.

CRYOTHERAPY

Lincoff first described the use of cryotherapy for treatment of intraocular tumors.[44,45] Only two primary choroidal melanomas were reported. Lincoff, in addition to having difficulty treating the entire lesion, also noted exudative retinal detachment and proliferative vitreoretinopathy following treatment. Histologic examination disclosed limited or no evidence of tumor destruction. However, others describe evidence that cryotherapy of small melanomas can produce tumor destruction.[1,2,7,10]

REFERENCES

1. Abramson DH, Ellsworth RM: Treatment of choroidal melanomas. Bull NY Acad Med 54:849-854, 1978.

2. Abramson DH, Lisman RD: Cryopexy of a choroidal melanoma. Ann Ophthalmol 11:1418-1421, 1979.

3. Apple DJ, Goldberg MF, Wyhinny G, Levi S: Argon laser photocoagulation of choroidal malignant melanoma. Arch Ophthalmol 90:97-101, 1973.

4. Astrahan M, Liggett P, Petrovich Z, Luxton G: A 500 kHz localized current field hyperthermia system for use with ophthalmic plaque radiotherapy. Int J Hyperthemia 3:423-432, 1987.

5. Barr CC, Norton EWD: Recurrence of choroidal melanoma after photocoagulation therapy. Arch Ophthalmol 101:1737-1740, 1983.

6. Boniuk M, Zimmerman LE: Occurrence and behavior of choroidal melanomas in eyes subjected to operations for retinal detachment. Tr Amer Acad Ophthalmol Oto 66:642-658, 1962.

7. Brovkina AF: Cryodestruction of choroidal melanomas. Vestn Oftalmol 2:61, 1977.

8. Bruce RA: Evaluation of hematoporphyrin photoradiation therapy to treat choroidal melanomas. Las Surg Med 4:59-64, 1984.

9. Burgess SEP, Chang S, Svitra P, et al.: Effect of hyperthermia on experimental choroidal melanoma. Br J Ophthalmol 69:854-860, 1985.

10. Char DH: The management of small choroidal melanomas. Surv Ophthalmol 22:377-386, 1978.

11. Char DH: Clinical Ocular Oncology. New York, Churchill-Livingstone, 1989, pp 91-149.

12. Coleman DJ, Lizzi FL, Burgess SEP, et al.: Ultrasonic hyperthermia and radiation in the management of intraocular malignant melanoma. Am J Ophthalmol 101:635-642, 1986.

13. Coleman DJ, Silverman RH, Iwamoto T, et al.: Histopathologic effects of ultrasonically induced hyperthermia in intraocular malignant melanoma. Ophthalmology 95:970-981, 1988.

14. Curtin VT, Norton EWD: Pathological changes in malignant melanomas after photocoagulation. Arch Ophthalmol 70:150-157, 1963.

15. Damato BE, Foulds WS: Ciliary body tumours and their management. Tr Ophthalmol Soc UK 105:257-264, 1986.

16. Davidorf FH, Newman GH, Havener WH, Makley T: Conservative management of malignant melanoma. II. Transscleral diathermy as a method of treatment for malignant melanoma of the choroid. Arch Ophthalmol 83:273-280, 1970.

17. De Laey JJ, Hanssens M, Ryckaert S: Photocoagulation of malignant melanomas of the choroid, a reappraisal. Bull Soc Belge Ophthalmol 213:9-18, 1986.

18. Dewey WC, Hopwood LE, Sapareto SA, Gerweck LE: Cellular responses to combinations of hyperthermia and radiation. Radiology 123:463-474, 1977.

19. Dougherty TJ, Kaufman JE, Goldfarb A, et al.: Photoradiation therapy for the treatment of malignant tumors. Canc Res 38:2628-2635, 1978.

20. Duvall J, Lucas DR: Argon laser and xenon arc coagulation of malignant choroidal melanomata: histological findings in 6 cases. Br J Ophthalmol 65:464-468, 1981.

21. Erie JC, Robertson DM: Serous detachments of the macula associated with presumed small choroidal melanomas. Am J Ophthalmol 102:176-178, 1986.

22. Finger PT, Packer S, Svitra PP, et al.: Hyperthermic treatment of intraocular tumors. Arch Ophthalmol 102:1477-1481, 1984.

23. Finger PT, Packer S, Svitra PP, et al.: Thermoradiotherapy for intraocular tumors. Arch Ophthalmol 103:1574-1578, 1985.

24. Folk JC, Weingeist TA, Coonan P, et al.: The treatment of serous macular detachment secondary to choroidal melanomas and nevi. Ophthalmology 96:547-551, 1989.

25. Foulds WS: The local excision of choroidal melanomata. Tr Ophthalmol Soc UK 93:343-346, 1973.

26. Foulds WS: Experience of local excision of uveal melanomas. Tr Ophthalmol Soc UK 97:412-415, 1977.

27. Foulds WS, Damato BE: Low-energy long-exposure laser therapy in the management of choroidal melanoma. Graefe's Arch Clin Exp Ophthalmol 224:26-31, 1986.

28. Francois J: Treatment of malignant melanoma of the choroid by light coagulation. Tr Ophthalmol Soc UK 85:179-189, 1965.

29. Francois J: Treatment of malignant melanoma of the choroid by light coagulation. Mod Probl Ophthalmol 12:550-555, 1974.

30. Francois J: Treatment of malignant choroidal melanomas by photocoagulation. Ophthalmologica 184:121-130, 1982.

31. Francois J: Disappearance of pigment after light coagulation of malignant melanoma of the choroid. Am J Ophthalmol 66:443-447, 1968.

32. Francois J: Treatment of malignant choroidal melanomas by xenon photocoagulation. In Lommatzsch PK, Blodi FC (eds): Intraocular Tumors. New York, Springer-Verlag, 1983, pp 277-285.

33. Francois J, De Laey JJ: Fluoro-angiography of photocoagulated malignant melanomas of the choroid. Mod Probl Ophthalmol 10:204-210, 1972.

34. Francois J, Hanssens M, De Laey JJ: Recurrence of malignant melanoma of the choroid seven and eight years after lightcoagulation. Ophthalmologica 162:188-192, 1971.

35. Fyodorov SN: The ablation of a choroidal melanoma. Ann Ophthalmol 4:510-513, 1972.

36. Gomer CJ, Doiron DR, Jester JV, et al.: Hematoporphyrin derivative photoradiation therapy for the treatment of intraocular tumors: examination of acute normal ocular tissue toxicity. Canc Res 43:721-727, 1983.

37. Hall EJ: Radiobiology For The Radiologist. Philadelphia, JB Lippincott, 1988, pp 27-35, 138-160, 162-177, 294-329.

38. Hepler RS, Allen RA, Straatsma BR: Photocoagulation of choroidal melanoma. Early and late histopathologic consequences. Arch Ophthalmol 79:177-181, 1968.

39. Kara GB: Excision of uveal melanomas: a 15-year experience. Tr Am Acad Ophthalmol Oto 86:997-1023, 1979.

40. Kim SH, Kim JH, Hahn EW: The radiosensitization of hypoxic tumor cells by hyperthermia. Radiology 114:727-730, 1975.

41. Kindy-Degnan N, Char DH, Swift P, et al.: Bromodeoxyuridine uptake in the assesment of hyperthermic therapy for intraocular tumor. Arch Ophthalmol 107:746-750, 1989.

42. Lagendijk JJW: A microwave heating technique for the hyperthermic treatment of tumors in the eye. Phys Med Biol 27:1313-1324, 1982.

43. Lewis RA, Tse DT, Phelps CE, Weingeist TA: Neovascular glaucoma after photoradiation therapy for uveal melanoma. Arch Ophthalmol 102:839-842, 1984.

44. Lincoff H: A report on the freezing of intraocular tumors. Mod Probl Ophthalmol 7:348-358, 1968.

45. Lincoff H, McLean J, Long R: The cryosurgical treatment of intraocular tumors. Am J Ophthalmol 63:389-399, 1967.

46. Lund OE: Histopathological changes in malignant melanoblastoma of the choroid after light-coagulation. Tr Ophthalmol Soc UK 84:99-105, 1964.

47. Lund OE: Changes in choroidal tumors after light coagulation (and diathermy coagulation). Arch Ophthalmol 75:458-466, 1966.

48. Makley TA, Havener WH, Newberg J: Light coagulation of intraocular tumors. Am J Ophthalmol 60:1082-1089, 1965.

49. Marmor JB, Pounds D, Postic TB, Hahn GM: Treatment of superficial human neoplasms by local hyperthermia induced by ultrasound. Cancer 43:188-197, 1979.

50. Meyer-Schwickerath G: Excision of malignant melanoma of the choroid. Mod Probl Ophthalmol 12:562-566, 1974.

51. Meyer-Schwickerath G: Photocoagulation of choroidal melanomas. Doc Ophthalmol 50:57-61, 1980.

52. Meyer-Schwickerath G: The preservation of vision by treatment of intraocular tumors with light coagulation. Arch Ophthalmol 66:458-466, 1961.

53. Meyer-Schwickerath G: Further progress in the field of light coagulation. Tr Ophthalmol Soc UK 77:421-440, 1957.

54. Meyer-Schwickerath G, Bornfeld N: Photocoagulation of choroidal melanomas - thirty years experience. In Lommatzsch PK, Blodi FC (Eds): Intraocular Tumors, New York, Springer-Verlag, 1983, pp 269-276.

55. Meyer-Schwickerath G, Vogel M: Treatment of malignant melanomas of the choroid by photocoagulation. Tr Ophthalmol Soc UK 97:416-420, 1977.

56. Meyer-Schwickerath G, Vogel MH: Malignant melanoma of the choroid treated with photocoagulation. A 10-year follow-up. Mod Probl Ophthalmol 12:544-549, 1974.

57. Mieler WF, Jaffe GJ, Steeves RA: Ferromagnetic hyperthermia and iodine 125 brachytherapy in the treatment of choroidal melanoma in a rabbit model. Arch Ophthalmol 107:1524-1528, 1989.

58. Naumann GOH, Volker HE, Gackle D: The blockexcision of malignant melanomas of the ciliary body and the peripheral choroid. Doc Ophthalmol 50:43-48, 1980.

59. Oosterhuis JA: Treatment of choroidal melanomas. Bull Soc Belge Ophthal 214:1-15, 1985.

60. Oosterhuis JA: Haematoporphyrin derivative photoradiation of malignant melanoma in the anterior chamber of the rabbit. In Oosterhuis JA (Ed): Ophthalmic Tumors. Dordrecht, Junk Publishers, 1985, pp 93-103.

61. Packer S: The management of choroidal melanoma. Arch Ophthalmol 102:1450-1451, 1984.

62. Peyman GA, Apple DJ: Local excision of a choroidal malignant melanoma. Full-thickness eye wall resection. Arch Ophthalmol 92:216-218, 1974.

63. Peyman GA, Axelrod AJ, Ericson ES, et al.: Full thickness eye wall resection in various species. An experimental approach in treatment of choroidal melanoma. Albrecht v Graefes Arch 186:157-164, 1973.

64. Peyman GA, Dodich NA: Full-thickness eye wall resection: an experimental approach for treatment of choroidal melanoma. I. Dacron-graft. Invest Ophthalmol 11:115-121, 1972.

65. Peyman GA, Ericson ES, Axelrod AJ, May DR: Full-thickness eye wall resection in primates. Arch Ophthalmol 89:410-412, 1973.

66. Peyman GA, Juarez CP, Diamond JG, Raichand M: Ten years experience with eye wall resection for uveal malignant melanomas. Ophthalmology 91:1720-1725, 1984.

67. Peyman GA, May DR, Ericson ES, Goldberg MF: Full-Thickness eye wall resection: An experimental approach for treatment of choroidal melanoma. II. Homo- and heterograft. Invest Ophthalmol 11:668-674, 1972.

68. Peyman GA, Raichand M, Schulman J: Diagnosis and therapeutic surgery of the uvea — part 1: Surgical technique. Ophthalmic Surg 17:822-829, 1986.

69. Peyman GA, Rednam KVR, Juarez CP: Improvement in eyewall resection technique. Ophthal Surg 14:588-591, 1983.

70. Peyman GA, Hindi M: Ab interno retinochoroidectomy in primates. Arch Ophthalmol 103:572-575, 1985.

71. Peyman GA, Charles H: Internal eye wall resection in the management of uveal melanoma. Can J Ophthalmol 23:219-223, 1988.

72. Pischel DK: Malignant melanoblastoma of the choroid. Results of treatment. Mod Probl Ophthalmol 7:84-85, 1968.

73. Riedel KG, Svitra PP, Seddon JM, et al.: Proton beam irradiation and hyperthermia. Arch Ophthalmol 103:1862-1869, 1985.

74. Ruiz RS: Early treatment in malignant melanomas of the choroid. In Brockhurst RJ, Boruchoff SA, Hutchinson BT, Lessel S (Eds): Controversy in Ophthalmology. Philadelphia, WB Saunders, 1977, pp 604-610.

75. Sautter H, Naumann G: Full-Thickness scleral resection in iridocyclectomy and choroidectomy for anterior uveal tumors. Ophthal Surg 4:25-31, 1973.

76. Sery TW, Dougherty TJ: Photoradiation of rabbit ocular malignant melanoma sensitized with hematoporphyrin derivative. Curr Eye Res 3:519-528, 1984.

77. Sery TW, Shields JA, Augsburger JJ, Shah HG: Photodynamic therapy of human ocular cancer. Ophthalmic Surg 18:413-418, 1987.

78. Shields JA: Changing trends in the management of choroidal melanomas. Tr Pac Coast Oto-Ophthalmol So 60:215-225, 1979.

79. Shields JA: Diagnosis And Management Of Intraocular Tumors. St. Louis, CV Mosby, 1983.

80. Shields JA, Glazer LC, Mieler WF, et al.: Comparison of xenon arc and argon laser photocoagulation in the treatment of choroidal melanomas. Am J Ophthalmol 109:647-655, 1990.

81. Shields JA, Shields CL: Surgical approach to lamellar sclerouvectomy for posterior uveal melanomas: The 1986 Schoenberg Lecture. Ophthalmic Surg 19:774-780, 1988.

82. Shukla M, Gerke E, Bornfeld N, Meyer-Schwickerath G: Tumor regression after photocoagulation of malignant melanomas of the choroid: an ultrasonographic study. Ophthalmologica 194:119-125, 1987.

83. Stallard HB: Pigmented tumours of the eye. Surgical aspects. Proc R Soc Lond 54:463-467, 1961.

84. Stallard HB: Partial choroidectomy. Br J Ophthalmol 50:660-662, 1966.

85. Tse DT, Dutton JJ, Weingeist TA, et al.: Hematoporphyrin photoradiation therapy for intraocular and orbital malignant melanoma. Arch Ophthalmol 102:833-838, 1984.

86. U R, Noell T, Woodward KT, et al.: Microwave-induced local hyperthermia in combination with radiotherapy of human malignant tumors. Cancer 45:638-646, 1980.

87. Vail DT: Iridocyclectomy. A review. Am J Ophthalmol 71:161-168, 1971.

88. Vogel MH: Xenon arc photocoagulation of small malignant melanomas of the choroid. In Peyman GA, Apple DJ, Saunders DR (Eds): Intraocular Tumors. New York, Appleton-Croft, 1977, pp 155-165.

89. Vogel MH: Histopathological observations of photocoagulated malignant melanomas of the choroid. Am J Ophthalmol 74:466-474, 1972.

90. Vogel MH: Treatment of malignant choroidal melanomas with photocoagulation. Evaluation of 10-year follow-up data. Am J Ophthalmol 74:1-11, 1972.

91. Vogel MH, Meyer-Schwickerath G: Results of photocoagulation treatment of malignant melanomas of the choroid. In Jakobiec F (Ed): Ocular and Adnexal Tumors. Birmingham, Aesculapius, 1978, pp 70-75.

92. Weve HJM: Diathermy in ophthalmic practice. Tr Ophthalmol Soc UK 59:61-64, 1939.

A FINAL PERSPECTIVE

Although significant advancements in the diagnosis and management of melanoma have occurred during the last several decades, there is still much to learn. In most cases, the diagnosis of malignant melanoma is not difficult, but important issues concerning smaller melanocytic lesions still must be resolved. Investigations of these concerns will certainly bring a better understanding of the tumor biology of malignant melanoma. Specifically, when does a small lesion need to be treated? When does metastasis occur? Presently, observed growth is the only available clinical parameter indicative of probable malignant potential. It is clear, however, that this is not completely satisfactory since clinically dormant lesions are rarely associated with metastatic disease. Conversely, does growth always indicate metastatic potential? And if so, how much growth? A clearer understanding of the likelihood of metastasis when a tumor grows is necessary. Developing more sensitive and specific indicators of metastatic disease and evaluating more and larger natural history studies may assist in resolving some of these questions.

Once a decision is made to treat, the optimal method is still not clear. This is most clearly evinced by the number of available treatment options. If the ideal treatment is defined as one that can achieve complete elimination or inactivation of malignant melanoma cells, survival of the patient, and retention of the eye with good vision, clearly no ideal treatment is available. Can an ideal treatment be developed? Which of the available methods is the best or least detrimental?

The Collaborative Ocular Melanoma Study is currently examining the relative merits of enucleation and [125]iodine plaque therapy. Recently, a study in the United Kingdom was begun examining proton beam irradiation compared with enucleation. The most important issue in studies involving malignant melanoma is which treatment maximizes survival. These studies should provide important data with which to counsel our patients.

Newer treatment modalities such as hyperthermia are promising, and may allow a reduction in the complications associated with radiation treatment. To date, experience with this technique is still preliminary. Finally, because newer treatment strategies have improved the prognosis of metastatic disease, is there a role for adjuvant chemotherapy in patients with certain high-risk tumors?

Only through earlier and more accurate diagnoses, better definition of the natural history, and improved treatment methods can Ophthalmology continue to affect significant improvements in the survival and treatment of patients with malignant melanoma.

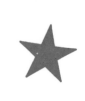